MRCGP
MULTIPLE CHOICE
REVISION BOOK

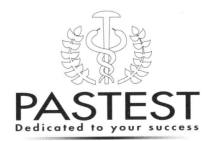

PASTEST
Dedicated to your success

© 2002 PasTest Ltd
Egerton Court
Parkgate Estate
Knutsford
Cheshire WA16 8DX

Telephone: 01565 752000

First edition 2002
Reprinted 2002

ISBN: 1 901198 55 3

A catalogue record for this book is available from the British Library.

The information contained within this book was obtained by the authors from
reliable sources. However, while every effort has been made to ensure its
accuracy, no responsibility for loss, damage or injury occasioned to any person
acting or refraining from action as a result of information contained herein can be
accepted by the publisher or the authors.

PasTest Revision Books and Intensive Courses

PasTest has been established in the field of postgraduate medical education
since 1972, providing revision books and intensive study courses for doctors
preparing for their professional examinations. Books and courses are available
for the following specialties:

**MRCGP, MRCP Part 1 and Part 2, MRCPCH Part 1 and Part 2, MRCOG,
DRCOG, MRCS, MRCPsych, DCH, FRCA and PLAB.**

For further details contact:

**PasTest Ltd, Freepost, Knutsford, Cheshire, WA16 7BR
Tel: 01565 752000   Fax: 01565 650264
Email: enquiries@pastest.co.uk   Web site: www. pastest.co.uk**

Typeset by Saxon Graphics Ltd, Derby
Printed by Bell and Bain Ltd, Glasgow

MRCGP MULTIPLE CHOICE REVISION BOOK

edited by

Peter Ellis MA MMed Ed MRCGP
Medical and Educational Advisor
London

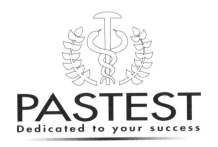

PASTEST
Dedicated to your success

CONTENTS

CONTRIBUTORS

DR R DANIELS   **MA MRCGP**
General Practitioner
Townsend House Medical Centre
Seaton
Devon

DR ANWAR A KHAN   **BSc MBBS DRCOG DCH (Lond) DCCH (Edin) FRCGP**
GP Trainer and course organiser
Loughton Health Centre
Loughton
Essex

and

Examiner
Royal College of General Practitioners

MAHENDRA MASHRU   **MSc MBBChir MRCS FRCGP**
General Practitioner
Ruislip
Middlesex

and

Honorary Senior Lecturer
Imperial College School of Medicine
London

INTRODUCTION

This Revision Book has been written to help candidates with their preparations for the Machine-marked paper of the MRCGP Examination. There are questions in various formats: Extended Matching Questions, Multiple Best Answer and Single Best Answer. All the questions are arranged by subject in sections which correspond with the headings published by the Royal College of General Practitioners in the information about the MRCGP Examination.

Candidates have indicated to us that they would like a book of questions sorted by subject, as they would find such an arrangement helpful when revising for this examination. We are always happy to receive comments about our material, and we would certainly like to know if this format has indeed been of help to you.

Good luck with the MRCGP Exam!

Peter Ellis
April 2002

MRCGP MEMBERSHIP EXAMINATION

The membership examination of the Royal College of General Practitioners is a constantly changing animal, and in the past it contained Multiple Choice Question papers, Modified Essay Question papers, Traditional Essay Questions and Practice Topic Questions.

The MRCGP Examination is now a modular examination consisting of four modules:

1. Written Paper – the examiner-marked paper
2. Multiple Choice Paper – the machine-marked paper
3. An assessment of consulting skills
4. Oral examination

To be successful in the MRCGP examination candidates must pass all four modules. There is a credit accumulation system and the modules can be taken together or at different sessions and can be taken in any order. This book is written for the machine-marked written paper: Paper 2, available twice a year.

The machine-marked paper is designed to test knowledge and application of that knowledge by candidates. From 2002 the paper will contain Extended Matching Questions (EMQ), Single Best Answer Questions (SBA), Multiple Best Answer Questions (MBA) and Summary Completion Questions (SCQ). All answers are recorded by candidates on sheets which can be machine-marked. The Royal College states that the number of items in each format is variable, and the maximum number of items in the paper will be 250. For the most up-to-date information, see the Royal College website at www.rcgp.org.uk

There is no negative marking for any of the question types in the machine marked written Module. There is therefore no point in leaving a question blank. It pays to guess! Questions are machine-scored on a basis of +1 mark for a correct answer and 0 for a wrong or missed response.

CONTENT OF THE MULTIPLE CHOICE PAPER

Medicine
- Cardiovascular
- Dermatology/ENT/Ophthalmology
- Endocrinology/Metabolic
- Gastroenterology/Nutrition
- Infectious diseases/Haematology/Immunology/Allergies/Genetics
- Paediatrics
- Pharmaco-therapeutics
- Psychiatry/Neurology
- Reproductive/Renal
- Respiratory

Administration and Management, including
- Regulatory framework of the NHS
- Legal aspects
- Business aspects
- Certification, benefits and allowances
- Professional regulation

Research, Epidemiology and Statistics, including
- Assessing the quality of care
- Principles of audit
- Understanding and application of the terms used in inferential statistics and evidence-based medicine
- Knowledge of statistics and research methodology, sufficient for the critical appraisal of published papers

EXAM PREPARATION AND TECHNIQUE

In trying to pass any examination it helps to plan an effective revision programme that concentrates on the elements that are being examined and not the areas which the exam cannot or does not test.

There are certain basic principles which are relevant to each part of the MRCGP exam.

i) Read relevant literature.
   Remember that this is an examination of British general practice. You will gain far more from reading a book about the consultation than from reading about ENT or ophthalmology etc in a textbook.

ii) Ask yourself WHY?
   The exam asks you to appraise critically what you are doing. After every consultation ask yourself about the outcome: did you feel happy about it, do you think the patient was satisfied with your management? If not, why not, and how could you have managed the situation better. After every article you read, ask yourself why the article was written, whether it was relevant, what the main points were that the author was trying to get across, and were there better ways of achieving the same result. Be critical in a constructive way about your work and your reading.

iii) Form an alliance with other candidates.
   By meeting on a regular basis you can stimulate one another to be more critical. You can also divide the onerous task of ploughing through journals between the group and become very much more knowledgeable very quickly. Finally, by talking to colleagues you will retain more factual knowledge and also be able to clarify your ideas and opinions more clearly.

There are also specific techniques which will help you to prepare for the machine-marked paper. It is often thought that you cannot improve your score in machine-marked examinations by repeatedly doing tests. We do not think that this is true. Candidates who do not improve their scores are using practice papers in the wrong way. What normally happens is that a candidate will spend a lot of time reading textbooks and then do a practice examination. It is far better to do an examination first, and then spend a lot of time reading around the answers and extending your knowledge in this way. Even with good teaching notes you still need to read around the topic.

There are only a limited number of areas relevant to general practice on which machine-marked questions can be set and by doing a number of practice examinations in this way you can substantially increase your knowledge base and thus increase your overall score.

ON EXAMINATION DAY

By the time the day of the examination arrives you will certainly have invested a good deal of money, and probably a lot of time and effort in the exam. It is important that you do not blow it all on the day by making silly mistakes.

Again there are certain basic rules for approaching each part of the MRCGP

i) Do not be tired.
   This may sound simple but if you have nights on call in the three to four days before the examination, then swap them. Try to keep your workload to a minimum. If you arrive tired you will not cope well with several hours of written work.

ii) Arrive in time.
   Every year, for both the written and oral examinations, candidates underestimate the time it will take them to get to the examination venue. They arrive distressed and anxious and under these circumstances can never do themselves justice.

iii) Key into the task.
   By arriving in plenty of time, you have the chance to prepare mentally for the examination. Reading a current journal quietly just before going into the exam will start your brain thinking about general practice and current issues. When you sit down to start working on the papers you will already be in the right frame of mind and this will save you valuable time.

iv) Read the instructions.
   No matter how well you think you know the rules, always read the instructions at the beginning. There should be no changes from previous years but just in case there are, this is time well spent.

The majority of candidates will not be short of time in the machine-marked paper, however there are a number of special techniques which should help:

i) Read the whole paper before you answer anything. This allows a lot of sub-conscious recall to happen before you start to mark your answers.

ii) Read every word in the stem and in each item. It is very easy to make simple mistakes by thinking that you read something that was not actually there.

iii) Mark the answer sheet carefully. Do not get the answer responses out of sequence. If you do have to alter a response rub it out well and mark the new response clearly. The answer sheets are marked by machine and an inadequately rubbed out answer could be interpreted as your true response.

iv) Answer every item. Remember there is NO negative marking and thus marks may be gained by guessing.

Finally, enjoy your studying using this book, and Good Luck with the Examination!

QUESTIONS

MEDICINE
QUESTIONS

CARDIOVASCULAR

EXTENDED MATCHING QUESTIONS

THEME: PULSES

A   Absent
B   Bisferiens
C   Collapsing
D   Pulsus paradoxus
E   Plateau
F   Pulsus alternans

For each of the descriptions, select the most likely type of pulse. Each option may be used once, more than once, or not at all.

1. Found in aortic stenosis ☐

2. Found in left ventricular failure ☐

3. Found in aortic regurgitation ☐

4. Found with mixed aortic stenosis and incompetence ☐

5. Usually noted when taking blood pressure – doubling in rate noted as mercury level falls ☐

6. Found with severe COPD ☐

7. Pulse volume decreases markedly with inspiration ☐

8. This is low amplitude with slow rise and fall ☐

THEME: ECG FINDINGS

A   Absent P waves with ragged baseline
B   Inverted T wave
C   Large R waves in V1–V2
D   Large S waves in V1–V2
E   Long QT interval
F   Peaked T wave
G   Prolonged PR interval
H   Short PR interval
I   Short QT interval

For each of the descriptions, select the most likely ECG finding. Each option may be used once, more than once, or not at all.

9. Wolff-Parkinson-White syndrome ☐

10. Atrial fibrillation ☐

11. Hyperkalaemia ☐

12. Right ventricular hypertrophy ☐

13. Hypercalcaemia ☐

14. 1st degree heart block ☐

15. Ischaemia or bundle branch block ☐

16. Hypocalcaemia ☐

17. Left ventricular hypertrophy ☐

MULTIPLE BEST ANSWER QUESTIONS

1. **A Mediterranean diet combines which TWO of the following?**
   - ☐ **A** Replaces poultry with red meat
   - ☐ **B** Increases fish, fruit and vegetables
   - ☐ **C** Reduces coronary artery disease more than just a low fat diet

2. **Adults who exercise regularly have which THREE of the following?**
   - ☐ **A** Lower blood pressure
   - ☐ **B** Increased risk of cancer of the colon
   - ☐ **C** Less likelihood of depression
   - ☐ **D** Less incidence of diabetes
   - ☐ **E** Improved co-ordination

3. **Select THREE items concerning cardiac rehabilitation after myocardial infarction**
   - ☐ **A** Can be carried out in General Practice
   - ☐ **B** Usually requires a clinical psychologist
   - ☐ **C** Needs to address diet and exercise
   - ☐ **D** Requires the use of beta-blockers and aspirin
   - ☐ **E** Is available to all patients in the UK

4. **In heart failure which THREE of the following have been shown to reduce mortality?**
   - ☐ **A** Thiazide diuretics
   - ☐ **B** Beta-blockers
   - ☐ **C** Digoxin
   - ☐ **D** Spironolactone
   - ☐ **E** ACE inhibitors

5. **Which THREE of the following statements are true of lipid lowering drugs?**
   - ☐ **A** Should be prescribed to a patient post MI with a cholesterol reading of 5.4
   - ☐ **B** Simvastatin is associated with sleep disturbance
   - ☐ **C** Should routinely be given to hypertensives with a cholesterol level > 7.8
   - ☐ **D** Are contraindicated in diabetes
   - ☐ **E** Compliance with statins is poor in some patients, due to gastro-intestinal side-effects

6. **Which TWO of the following drugs should be avoided in hypertensive patients with the following conditions?**
   - ☐ **A** Thiazide diuretics in patients with gout
   - ☐ **B** Calcium antagonists in patients with glucose intolerance
   - ☐ **C** Beta-blockers in patients with obstructive airways disease

7. **Select THREE statements concerning events following myocardial infarction**

- ☐ **A** 50% of deaths occur within two hours of onset of symptoms
- ☐ **B** Ventricular fibrillation is most likely to occur at 48–72 hours
- ☐ **C** The ECG can remain normal for several hours
- ☐ **D** The ECG can remain normal for several days
- ☐ **E** Thrombolytic therapy is contraindicated until chest pain has resolved

8. **Which TWO of the following statements about angina pectoris are correct?**

- ☐ **A** May occur with normal coronary arteries
- ☐ **B** Is associated with abnormal resting ECG between attacks in about 90% of cases
- ☐ **C** Is typically worse later in the day
- ☐ **D** ST segment elevation on ECG is usual during an attack
- ☐ **E** May be aggravated by lying down

9. **Select THREE of the following statements concerning deep venous thrombosis**

- ☐ **A** Is not common in patients over the age of 40
- ☐ **B** Has been linked to long-haul flights
- ☐ **C** Varicose veins are a recognised risk factor
- ☐ **D** Oral combined contraceptive pill should be stopped before major surgery
- ☐ **E** Calf vein thrombosis should be treated with heparin

SINGLE BEST ANSWER QUESTIONS

1. Select ONE of these statements regarding the management of hypertension

- ☐ **A** The therapeutic target in a diabetic is <130/85
- ☐ **B** Beta-blockers are contraindicated in gout
- ☐ **C** Thiazide diuretics should not be first-line in type 1 diabetes
- ☐ **D** Isolated systolic hypertension in a 79-year-old requires treatment
- ☐ **E** In 66% of hypertensives, optimal readings can be achieved using monotherapy

2. A high mortality following myocardial infarction is NOT associated with which ONE of the following

- ☐ **A** Increasing age
- ☐ **B** High blood pressure
- ☐ **C** High heart rate on admission to hospital
- ☐ **D** Anterior infarction pattern on ECG
- ☐ **E** Previous infarction

3. Select ONE of the following statements about angioplasty

- ☐ **A** Is ideal for treatment of discrete stenosis of the main stem of the left coronary artery
- ☐ **B** Is dangerous for patients with multiple vessel disease
- ☐ **C** Is contraindicated in patients who have undergone bypass surgery
- ☐ **D** Is contraindicated in patients with unstable angina
- ☐ **E** May involve complications if there is acute occlusion of the lesion

DERMATOLOGY/ ENT PROBLEMS/ OPTHALMOLOGY

DERMATOLOGY

EXTENDED MATCHING QUESTIONS

THEME: RASHES

A Dermatitis artefacta
B Dermatitis herpetiformis
C Lichen simplex
D Nodular prurigo

For each of the descriptions, select the most likely rash. Each option may be used once, more than once, or not at all.

1. This rash characteristically has straight sides ☐

2. If the itch/scratch cycle is interrupted then this lichenified rash disappears ☐

3. This rash affects young adults. It is an itchy, vesicular rash with psoriatic distribution. ☐

4. This rash on the hands heals to leave white scars with follicular openings in them ☐

THEME: CAUSES OF NAIL DISCOLORATION

A Chloroquine
B Leuconychia
C Penicillamine
D Tinea infection
E Trauma
F Yellow nail syndrome

For each description below, select the single most likely option. Each option may be used once, more than once, or not at all.

5. The nail is curved longitudinally and transversally and is associated with lymphoedema ☐

6. The nails are stained yellow after taking certain medication ☐

7. The nails are stained blue-grey ☐

8. This is inherited as an autosomal dominant gene ☐

9. The nails often have white streaks ☐

10. There are yellow thickened areas with slow growth of the nail ☐

11. The whole nail is white ☐

THEME: RASHES

A Erythema multiforme
B Ichthyosis
C Infected eczema
D Pustular psoriasis
E Scabies

For each description below, select the single most likely option. Each option may be used once, more than once, or not at all.

12. This rash has secondary staphylococcal infection ☐

13. There is scaly dry skin on the fingers ☐

14. A large vesicle with a surrounding red halo is characteristic ☐

15. Lesions are often seen on the soles of the feet and palms of the hand ☐

16. Burrows occur on the sides of the fingers ☐

THEME: SKIN CONDITIONS

A   Plaque psoriasis
B   Irritant contact dermatitis
C   Guttate psoriasis
D   Allergic contact dermatitis
E   Atopic dermatitis
F   Pompholyx
G   Seborrhoeic dermatitis
H   Asteatotic eczema
I   Erythrodermic psoriasis
J   Pustular psoriasis

For each of the descriptions below, select the most appropriate diagnosis from the list above. Each option may be used once, more than once, or not at all.

17. Most commonly seen in children and adolescents, there are numerous small scaly papules and plaques ☐

18. Follows repeated exposure to an irritant e.g. mineral oils in motor mechanics ☐

19. An eruption of vesicles on the sides of fingers, palms or soles of feet, which may be extremely itchy ☐

20. Also known as Red Man Syndrome, this skin disease may affect the whole body and lead to hypothermia, hypoproteinaemia and high output heart failure ☐

21. An erythematous condition, often with scaling in a characteristic crazy-paving pattern, seen on the shins of the elderly ☐

THEME: LEG ULCERS

A   Ischaemic ulcers
B   Venous ulcers

For each description, select the most likely type of leg ulcer. Each option may be used once, more than once, or not at all.

22. Usually have marked induration and oedema ☐

23. Usually painless and pigmented ☐

24. Tend to be punched out and necrotic ☐

25. Are painful and most frequently seen in elderly people ☐

26. The surrounding skin may be eczematous ☐

MULTIPLE BEST ANSWER QUESTIONS

1. **Which THREE of the following nail signs are suggestive of the associated conditions?**
    - ☐ **A** Transverse grooves and psoriasis
    - ☐ **B** Opaque nails and diabetes mellitus
    - ☐ **C** Splinter haemorrhages and bacterial endocarditis
    - ☐ **D** Blue nails and pseudomonas spp. infection
    - ☐ **E** Green nails and lichen planus

2. **Which TWO of the following skin conditions generally deteriorate during pregnancy?**
    - ☐ **A** Atopic eczema
    - ☐ **B** Systemic lupus erythematosus
    - ☐ **C** Hidradenitis suppurativa
    - ☐ **D** Herpes simplex

3. **Which TWO of the following drugs are characteristically linked with the following type of reaction?**
    - ☐ **A** Oral contraceptives and photosensitivity
    - ☐ **B** Codeine and urticaria
    - ☐ **C** Tetracycline and exfoliative dermatitis
    - ☐ **D** Fucidin and pigmentation
    - ☐ **E** Beta-blockers and eczema

4. **Select THREE items which are true of Granuloma annulare**
    - ☐ **A** Is more common on the trunk
    - ☐ **B** Is painful
    - ☐ **C** Is associated with diabetes
    - ☐ **D** May persist for many years
    - ☐ **E** Lacks effective treatment

5. **Which TWO of the following conditions are associated with erythema nodosum?**
    - ☐ **A** Herpes simplex
    - ☐ **B** Tuberculosis
    - ☐ **C** Inflammatory bowel disease
    - ☐ **D** Hyperthyroidism

6. **Which TWO of the following drugs may precipitate or exacerbate psoriasis?**
    - ☐ **A** Lithium
    - ☐ **B** Hydralazine
    - ☐ **C** H_2-antagonists
    - ☐ **D** Beta-blockers
    - ☐ **E** Anticonvulsants

7. Select THREE of the following items concerning alopecia areata

- ☐ **A**   Is a scarring process with permanent loss of follicles
- ☐ **B**   Is associated with auto-immune thyroid disease
- ☐ **C**   Is confined to scalp hairs
- ☐ **D**   Is a recognised association of Down's syndrome
- ☐ **E**   May be associated with nail changes

8. Select THREE of the following statements about acne vulgaris

- ☐ **A**   Most teenagers with acne seek treatment for it
- ☐ **B**   The key pathological event in acne is obstruction of the pilosebaceous duct
- ☐ **C**   The severity of acne is directly related to the degree of secretion of sebum
- ☐ **D**   Circulating levels of androgen are usually high in patients with acne
- ☐ **E**   An open comedo (blackhead) results from the rupture of the wall of the pilo-sebaceous duct and release of the contents in the dermis

SINGLE BEST ANSWER QUESTIONS

1. **Select ONE of the following regarding basal cell carcinoma**
   - ☐ **A** The most common skin malignancy in Caucasians
   - ☐ **B** Almost never occurs on covered skin sites
   - ☐ **C** Should no longer be treated by curettage and cautery since results are inferior to other treatment methods

2. **Select ONE of the following regarding multiple seborrhoeic warts**
   - ☐ **A** Most commonly found on the face and trunk
   - ☐ **B** Usually infective
   - ☐ **C** Best removed by excision

3. **The ONE most recognised cause of erythema nodosum from the list below is**
   - ☐ **A** Sarcoidosis
   - ☐ **B** Oral contraceptives
   - ☐ **C** Preceding mycoplasmal infection

4. **You see a 6-year-old child in surgery with his mother. He has been diagnosed with molluscum contagiosum and she is keen to have them treated. Which ONE of the following is true?**
   - ☐ **A** The condition resolves spontaneously
   - ☐ **B** The condition is not infectious
   - ☐ **C** Patients may treat themselves by squeezing the spots with no adverse effects
   - ☐ **D** It is only seen in children
   - ☐ **E** Piercing the lesions with an orange stick dipped in phenol is the treatment of choice

5. **You are setting up a leg ulcer clinic to be run by your practice nurse. Which ONE of the following is the single best treatment for venous leg ulcers?**
   - ☐ **A** Aspirin
   - ☐ **B** Compression bandaging
   - ☐ **C** Zinc paste
   - ☐ **D** Intermittent pneumatic calf compression
   - ☐ **E** Hyperbaric oxygen

ENT PROBLEMS

EXTENDED MATCHING QUESTIONS

THEME: LESIONS ON THE EAR

A Chilblains
B Kerato-acanthoma
C Psoriatic
D Rodent ulcer
E Squamous cell cancer
F Tophi

For each of the descriptions, select the single most likely lesion. Each option may be used once, more than once, or not at all.

1. These lesions are common, painful and itchy ☐

2. This is a slow growing lesion found on the helix ☐

3. These lesions are usually found on the antihelix ☐

4. These lesions are rapidly growing and usually found on the helix ☐

5. These lesions are found usually behind and below the ear ☐

6. These lesions are found in the external auditory meatus and on the skin behind and below the ear ☐

THEME: HOARSENESS

A Diabetes mellitus
B Gastro-oesophageal reflux
C Myxoedema
D Pharyngeal neoplasia
E Smoking
F Thyrotoxicosis

For each patient with hoarseness, select the single most likely diagnosis. Each option can be used once, more than once or not at all.

7. Hoarseness with weight loss

8. Hoarseness in otherwise healthy adult

9. Hoarseness with weight gain

10. Hoarseness with associated dysphagia

11. Hoarseness with dyspepsia

THEME: EARACHE

A   Otitis media
B   Otitis externa
C   Tonsillitis
D   Glue Ear
E   Meniere's disease
F   Tonsillar carcinoma
G   Furuncle
H   Bullous haemorrhagic myringitis
I   Ramsay Hunt syndrome
J   Cerebello-pontine angle tumours

For each of the descriptions below, select the most appropriate diagnosis from the list above. Each option may be used once, more than once or not at all.

12. Earache associated with imbalance, deafness and vesicles in the ear canal ☐

13. Peak incidence is around 6 years old, this condition is the commonest cause of conductive hearing loss ☐

14. Should be considered in patients with unilateral tinnitus, unsteadiness and deafness ☐

15. May present with diarrohoea and vomiting in young children ☐

16. May be caused by hearing aids ☐

MULTIPLE BEST ANSWER QUESTIONS

1. Glue ear is commonly associated with which TWO of the following?
- ☐ **A** Atopy
- ☐ **B** Neomycin treatment
- ☐ **C** Breast-fed babies compared with bottle-fed
- ☐ **D** Meningitis
- ☐ **E** Down's syndrome

2. Which THREE of the following predispose to oral cancer?
- ☐ **A** High alcohol consumption
- ☐ **B** Smoking cigarettes
- ☐ **C** Folate deficiency
- ☐ **D** Tea drinking
- ☐ **E** Cigar smoking

3. Which THREE of the following factors pre-dispose to otitis externa?
- ☐ **A** Ear syringing
- ☐ **B** Under 5-year-olds
- ☐ **C** Diabetes mellitus
- ☐ **D** Psoriasis
- ☐ **E** Diving

4. Which THREE of the following drugs cause a dry mouth?
- ☐ **A** Monoamine oxidase inhibitors
- ☐ **B** Antihistamines
- ☐ **C** Bronchoconstrictors
- ☐ **D** Phenothiazines
- ☐ **E** Amphetamines

SINGLE BEST ANSWER QUESTIONS

1. **Which ONE of the following is a recognised cause of conductive deafness in children?**
    - ☐ **A** Glue ear
    - ☐ **B** Post-meningitis
    - ☐ **C** Congenital rubella
    - ☐ **D** Mumps
    - ☐ **E** Kernicterus

2. **You see a 29-year-old policeman in surgery who complains of mild allergic rhinitis. Which ONE of the following is the best initial treatment?**
    - ☐ **A** Referral for RAST testing for common allergens
    - ☐ **B** Oral desloratadine
    - ☐ **C** Nasal fluticasone on a prn basis
    - ☐ **D** Reduction in house dust mite exposure
    - ☐ **E** Chlorpheniramine
    - ☐ **F** Regular Xylometolazone

3. **A 72-year-old man is brought to see you by his wife who says she is sick of having to shout every time she wants to talk to him. An audiogram confirms sensorineural deafness. Which ONE of the following is the likeliest cause?**
    - ☐ **A** Otosclerosis
    - ☐ **B** Multiple sclerosis
    - ☐ **C** Barotrauma
    - ☐ **D** Presbyacusis
    - ☐ **E** Menière's disease

OPHTHALMOLOGY

EXTENDED MATCHING QUESTIONS

THEME: SUDDEN LOSS OF VISION

A Central retinal vein occlusion
B Migraine
C Optic neuritis
D Senile macular degeneration
E Toxic optic neuropathy

For each description, select the single most likely cause of sudden loss of vision. Each option may be used once, more than once, or not at all.

1. There is a gradual loss of vision in people between 20 and 45 years old. The peripheral vision is intact. ☐

2. There is a gradually progressive loss of vision in an older person. There is preservation of peripheral fields. ☐

3. This tends to occur in heavy cigarette smokers. Peripheral vision remains largely intact. ☐

4. There is complete recovery from this loss of vision which often, but not always, occurs with headache. ☐

5. There is extensive haemorrhage visible at the fundus. Visual loss develops over a few hours. ☐

THEME: RED EYE

A   Acute glaucoma
B   Episcleritis
C   Iritis
D   Keratitis
E   Sub-conjunctival haemorrhage

For each description, select the single most likely cause of red eye. Each option may be used once, more than once, or not at all.

6. This is associated with impaired vision. An ulcer may be found near the visual axis. ☐

7. There is slight or no pain. Vision tends to be normal and the red eye will settle without treatment. ☐

8. The pupil is small but often distorted. ☐

9. There is severe pain with severe visual impairment. Vomiting commonly occurs. ☐

10. This red eye is painless and vision is normal. ☐

THEME: VISUAL FIELD DEFECTS

A Arcuate scotoma
B Central scotoma
C Centrocaecal scotoma
D Ring scotoma

For each description, select the single most likely cause of visual field defect. Each option may be used once, more than once, or not at all.

11. This is characteristic of glaucoma ☐

12. This field defect occurs in toxic neuropathy ☐

13. This scotoma is typical of retinitis pigmentosa ☐

14. This defect is characteristic of disease affecting the macula ☐

THEME: EYE LESIONS

A Corneal arcus
B Kayser-Fleischer rings
C Pinguecula
D Pterygium
E Sub-conjunctival haemorrhage

For each description, select the single most likely cause of an eye lesion. Each option may be used once, more than once, or not at all.

15. A triangular fold of conjunctiva found between the canthus and the corneal edge ☐

16. A white ring found near the outer margin of the cornea ☐

17. A bright red mark seen on the conjunctiva ☐

18. A yellowish brown deposit seen at the periphery of the cornea ☐

19. A yellow deposit noted between the canthus and the edge of the cornea ☐

20. Due to a deposit of copper ☐

21. May occur as a result of whooping cough or labour ☐

MULTIPLE BEST ANSWER QUESTIONS

1. **Select TWO of the following list as features of acute iritis**
   - ☐ **A** Dilated pupil
   - ☐ **B** Circumcorneal redness
   - ☐ **C** Blurred vision
   - ☐ **D** Purulent discharge
   - ☐ **E** Eye hard and tender

2. **Select TWO visual findings in myopia**
   - ☐ **A** Minus (concave) lenses are required in the ophthalmoscope to view the fundus
   - ☐ **B** The optic disc may look small
   - ☐ **C** The optic disc may look particularly bright
   - ☐ **D** There may be surrounding chorioretinal atrophy

3. **Select FOUR of the following statements about visual fundus findings**
   - ☐ **A** Hard exudates are caused by sugars leaking out of blood vessels
   - ☐ **B** Hard exudates are seen in diabetes and hypertension
   - ☐ **C** Hard exudates look like deposits of cotton wool
   - ☐ **D** Soft exudates are due to swelling of the axons in the nerve fibre layer
   - ☐ **E** Soft exudates are well defined yellow white deposits, often in rings
   - ☐ **F** Soft exudates occur around an area of infarcted retina
   - ☐ **G** Soft exudates are often associated with features of retinal ischaemia such as new blood vessel formation

SINGLE BEST ANSWER QUESTIONS

1. **What is the commonest cause of blindness over the age of 65 years?**
   - ☐ **A** Glaucoma
   - ☐ **B** Cataract
   - ☐ **C** Diabetic retinopathy
   - ☐ **D** Macular degeneration

2. **What is the commonest cause of blindness in people age 45–64?**
   - ☐ **A** Diabetic retinopathy
   - ☐ **B** Macular degeneration
   - ☐ **C** Glaucoma
   - ☐ **D** Optic atrophy

3. **Cataracts are NOT usually associated with**
   - ☐ **A** myotonic dystrophy
   - ☐ **B** thyrotoxicosis
   - ☐ **C** diabetes mellitus
   - ☐ **D** rubella
   - ☐ **E** hyperparathyroidism

4. **Select ONE statement. Diabetic maculopathy**
   - ☐ **A** is more common in NIDDM than IDDM
   - ☐ **B** impairs peripheral vision
   - ☐ **C** is treated by pan-retinal photocoagulation
   - ☐ **D** is characterised by drusen at the macula
   - ☐ **E** causes painful visual loss

5. **A patient presents with a painful red eye. Which ONE of the following findings is more suggestive of acute conjunctivitis than anterior uveitis?**
   - ☐ **A** Blurring of vision
   - ☐ **B** Profuse discharge
   - ☐ **C** Small pupil
   - ☐ **D** Photophobia

ENDOCRINOLOGY/ METABOLIC

EXTENDED MATCHING QUESTIONS

THEME: ENDOCRINE DISEASES

A Acromegaly
B Conn's
C Cushing's
D Diabetes insipidus
E Simmond's

For each of the descriptions, select the most likely endocrine disease. Each option may be used once, more than once, or not at all.

1. Caused by excess growth hormone ☐

2. Caused by a deficiency of ADH ☐

3. Associated with excess corticosteroid ☐

4. Associated with excess aldosterone ☐

5. Associated with deficiencies of growth hormone, FSH and LH ☐

THEME: METABOLIC BONE DISEASE

A Hyperparathyroidism
B Hypoparathyroidism
C Osteomalacia
D Osteoporosis
E Paget's
F Renal osteodystrophy
G Rickets

For each of the descriptions, select the most likely metabolic bone disease. Each option may be used once, more than once, or not at all.

6. Associated with a greatly increased alkaline phosphatase level, bone pain and tenderness. The sacrum and lumbar spine are the bones most commonly affected. □

7. Children present with leg and chest deformities. It is associated with increased alkaline phosphatase and decreased phosphate levels. □

8. Presents with bone pain and tenderness and is associated with a moderate increase in alkaline phosphatase levels, decreased phosphate and calcium levels. □

9. Associated with decreased calcium levels but increased phosphate levels. □

10. This disease can be complicated by progressive occlusion of skull foramina causing deafness, and also by high output cardiac failure. □

11. Associated with increased calcium levels, bone cysts and sub-periosteal erosions in the phalanges. □

12. This gives cupping, splaying and fraying of the epiphyses. □

13. Hormone replacement therapy is given to try to avoid this disease. □

THEME: ARTHRITIS

A Primary nodal osteoarthritis
B Rheumatoid arthritis
C Psoriatic arthritis
D Dysbaric osteonecrosis
E Septic arthritis
F Systemic Lupus Erythematosus
G Gout
H Ankylosing spondylitis
I Reiter's syndrome
J Rheumatic fever
K Pseudogout
L Rubella

Read the case summaries below and select the most appropriate diagnosis from the list above. Each option may be used once, more than once or not at all.

14. A 37-year-old man with several year history of backache, which disturbs his sleep. He has early morning stiffness, which improves with exercise.

15. A 19-year-old sewage worker presents with bilateral knee pain and stiffness. He also mentions red spots on his feet that are turning into pustules. These symptoms started a few days after an episode of gastroenteritis.

16. A 45-year-old accountant complains of recurrent pain in the ends of his fingers and toes. He tells you that it seems to get worse when his skin is dry and he has thickened distorted nails on the affected fingers.

17. A 21-year-old woman presents with fever and rigors. She has also developed a swollen, red and painful knee.

18. A 44-year-old man with mild hypertension, recently started on diuretics, wakes up in the middle of the night with severe pain in his big toe. On examination the skin overlying the joint is red, swollen and warm.

19. A 4-year-old child who has been unwell for several days with coryzal symptoms and conjunctivitis develops a rash, initially on his face but spreading to his trunk. He subsequently complains of pain and stiffness in his metacarpophalangeal and proximal interphalangeal joints.

MULTIPLE BEST ANSWER QUESTIONS

1. Choose THREE statements about gout
- [ ] **A**   Predominantly affects males
- [ ] **B**   Is usually, but not always, accompanied by elevated serum uric acid levels
- [ ] **C**   Is associated with high alcohol intake, due to the high purine content of alcoholic drinks
- [ ] **D**   Is closely associated with potassium-sparing diuretics
- [ ] **E**   Can cause renal impairment

2. Select THREE features of osteoporosis
- [ ] **A**   The WHO defines osteoporosis as a bone density of one standard deviation below the mean
- [ ] **B**   More than 30% of women will have an osteoporotic fracture
- [ ] **C**   More than 10% of men will sustain an osteoporotic fracture
- [ ] **D**   Bone density starts to fall at the age of 40 years
- [ ] **E**   Bone densitometry helps to identify those women who will sustain a fracture

3. Select TWO features of Wilson's disease
- [ ] **A**   Is inherited as an autosomal dominant
- [ ] **B**   Is a disorder of iron metabolism
- [ ] **C**   Often presents with polyarthropathy
- [ ] **D**   Can result in cirrhosis from depositions in the liver
- [ ] **E**   Is associated with choreoathetosis
- [ ] **F**   Is commonly associated with diabetes

4. Select TWO of these items about the treatment of non-insulin dependent diabetes (NIDDM)
- [ ] **A**   Insulin resistance contributes to the hyperglycaemia
- [ ] **B**   Glibenclamide is safer than glipizide in the elderly
- [ ] **C**   Metformin frequently causes hypoglycaemia
- [ ] **D**   Chlorpropamide may cause facial flushing

5. Hyperuricaemia may be induced by which THREE of the following?
- [ ] **A**   Frusemide
- [ ] **B**   Polycythaemia rubra vera
- [ ] **C**   Myxoedema
- [ ] **D**   Multiple myeloma
- [ ] **E**   Diabetes mellitus

6. TWO known risk factors for osteoporosis are
- [ ] **A**   History of alcoholism
- [ ] **B**   Oral steroid treatment
- [ ] **C**   Myxoedema
- [ ] **D**   Late menopause

7. **Select THREE of the following statements about haemochromatosis**

☐ **A**   Is inherited as an autosomal recessive
☐ **B**   Is a disorder of copper metabolism
☐ **C**   Often presents with diabetes
☐ **D**   Is often associated with skin pigmentation
☐ **E**   May present with hepatomegaly
☐ **F**   May result in Kayser-Fleischer rings in the eyes

8. **Which of the following THREE conditions are recognised causes of fasting hypoglycaemia**

☐ **A**   Lung cancer
☐ **B**   Alcoholism
☐ **C**   Addison's disease
☐ **D**   Hepatic carcinoma
☐ **E**   Chronic gout
☐ **F**   Myxoedema

9. **THREE recognised complications in pregnancies of diabetic women are**

☐ **A**   Oligohydramnios
☐ **B**   Pre-eclampsia
☐ **C**   Congenital abnormalities
☐ **D**   Intra-uterine growth retardation
☐ **E**   Intra-uterine death

SINGLE BEST ANSWER QUESTIONS

1.   Which ONE of the following does NOT occur in hypothyroidism?

☐   **A**   Carpal tunnel syndrome
☐   **B**   Pretibial myxoedema
☐   **C**   Macrocytosis
☐   **D**   A normal serum triiodothyronine (T_3) concentration

2.   Carpal tunnel syndrome is not usually associated with which ONE of the following?

☐   **A**   Pregnancy
☐   **B**   Rheumatoid arthritis
☐   **C**   Thyrotoxicosis
☐   **D**   Previous scaphoid fracture
☐   **E**   Acromegaly

GASTROENTEROLOGY/ NUTRITION

EXTENDED MATCHING QUESTIONS

THEME: CAUSES OF ABDOMINAL PAIN

A   Crohn's disease
B   Irritable bowel syndrome
C   Diverticular disease
D   Ischaemic colitis
E   Pancreatitis
F   Cholecystitis
G   Appendicitis

For each of the following scenarios, select the most appropriate option. Each option may be used once, more than once, or not at all.

1. A 41-year-old restaurant manager who has severe abdominal pain radiating to his back.

2. A 72-year-old lady who has 'life-long' constipation and has had vague abdominal pain for months or even years. She is tender in her left lower abdomen.

3. A 31-year-old doctor who has abdominal pain relieved by defaecation, she has frequent loose motions often after meals. She is tender over her sigmoid colon.

4. A 69-year-old lady with abdominal pain and bloody diarrhoea. She has frequent angina. Her abdomen is generally tender.

5. A 58-year-old female teacher with feelings of 'fullness' and alternating diarrhoea and constipation. The pain is often relieved by passing platus. She is tender in the left iliac fossa.

6. A 49-year-old architect who has abdominal pain that he finds difficult to place, but says it is severe at times. His abdomen is generally tender especially over the upper quadrants.

7. A 41-year-old librarian with abdominal pain and diarrhoea. His abdomen is generally tender and he is noted to have anal tags.

THEME: CHANGE IN BOWEL HABIT

A   Toddler diarrhoea
B   Laxative abuse
C   Ulcerative colitis
D   Viral gastroenteritis
E   Crohn's disease
F   Colon cancer
G   Coeliac disease
H   Carcinoid syndrome
I   Giardiasis
J   Irritable Bowel Syndrome
K   Hyperthyroidism

For each of the scenarios described below, pick the single most likely diagnosis. Each answer may be used once, more than once or not at all.

8. The patient is systemically well. Stools often contain undigested food, such as peas or carrots. ☐

9. Typically presents in the third to fourth decade with altered bowel habit, pain and bloating. Commoner in women than men, symptoms do not usually disturb sleep. ☐

10. Causes bloody diarrhoea , up to 10 times a day. Relapses may be associated with stopping smoking. ☐

11. Characteristically causes flushing provoked by stress or alcohol. The diarrhoea is associated with weight loss, dyspnoea and wheezing. ☐

12. May be associated with increased appetite, palpitations, weight loss, anxiety and sweating. ☐

13. May present in childhood as failure to thrive, or in adults with diarrhoea, lethargy and malaise. May have an associated itchy vesicular rash. ☐

14. Characterised by an acute onset of anorexia, nausea, abdominal distension and frequent frothy yellow offensive stools. ☐

THEME: INDIGESTION

A   H$_2$ receptor antagonist
B   Proton pump inhibitor
C   Alginates
D   Nissan's fundoplication
E   Cisapride
F   Domperidone
G   Triple therapy
H   Misoprostol
I   Calcium carbonate

For each of the clinical situations described below, select the most appropriate treatment from the list above. Each option may be used once, more than once or not at all.

15. The first-line treatment for reflux in pregnancy

16. Should be considered in patients shown to have erosive oesophagitis on endoscopy

17. May be used in combination with NSAIDs to prevent ulcer formation

18. Should be considered for refractory reflux disease

19. The first-line treatment for H. pylori positive patients with reflux symptoms, whose symptoms are not helped by alginates

MULTIPLE BEST ANSWER QUESTIONS

1. **Select TWO of the following statements about gallstones**
   - ☐ **A** Cholesterol stones are strongly associated with bacteria in the bile
   - ☐ **B** The incidence of stones in the gall bladder rises with age
   - ☐ **C** Few stones remain symptomless
   - ☐ **D** Treatment with chenodeoxycholic acid may be effective for pigment stones
   - ☐ **E** Cholecystectomy is the standard treatment for symptomatic gallstones

2. **Select TWO of the following items concerning *Helicobacter pylori***
   - ☐ **A** Infection is usually acquired in the first 5 years of life
   - ☐ **B** Is found in 50% of those over 50 years in developed countries
   - ☐ **C** Is strongly associated with gastro-oesophageal reflux
   - ☐ **D** Infection rate is increasing with improved socio-economic conditions
   - ☐ **E** Breath test remains positive for about six months after eradication treatment

3. **Select TWO of the following items about acute gastroenteritis**
   - ☐ **A** Patients with an ileostomy are at increased risk from dehydration
   - ☐ **B** Refeeding should commence as soon as the appetite returns
   - ☐ **C** Oral rehydration therapy (ORT) improves the diarrhoea
   - ☐ **D** Antibiotics are contraindicated with Campylobacter infection
   - ☐ **E** Commercial ORT is inadequate for children <2 years of age

4. **Which TWO of the following are recognised complications of Crohn's disease?**
   - ☐ **A** Small bowel obstruction
   - ☐ **B** Clubbing
   - ☐ **C** Polycythaemia
   - ☐ **D** Thrombophlebitis
   - ☐ **E** Amyloidosis

5. **Select TWO of these statements about peptic ulceration**
   - ☐ **A** Is associated with H. pylori infection in >90% of the cases
   - ☐ **B** Endoscopy is an essential diagnostic test
   - ☐ **C** In case of duodenal ulceration, pain is related to hunger
   - ☐ **D** Vomiting associated with pain is a diagnostic feature
   - ☐ **E** H_2-antagonists have a place in the treatment

6. **Select TWO of the following statements about duodenal ulceration**
   - ☐ **A** Usually occurs in the duodenal bulb
   - ☐ **B** Affects approximately 10% of the population
   - ☐ **C** Has been proved to be caused by non-steroidal anti-inflammatory drugs
   - ☐ **D** Has a natural history of settling spontaneously within 5–10 years of onset
   - ☐ **E** Causes pain with a characteristic history of occurring immediately after food

7. **In cancer of the colon, which THREE statements apply?**
    ☐ **A** The overall 5-year survival rate is now about 50%
    ☐ **B** There is an increased risk in patients with inflammatory bowel disease
    ☐ **C** There is greater risk in patients with a family history of non polyposis colonic cancer
    ☐ **D** There is an increased risk in patients who have two first-degree relatives with colonic cancer
    ☐ **E** Screening for faecal occult blood has a high sensitivity but a low specificity

8. **Select THREE statements concerning diverticular disease of the colon**
    ☐ **A** Is less common in vegetarians
    ☐ **B** Is commonly limited to the sigmoid colon
    ☐ **C** In General Practice, change in bowel habit is the most common presentation
    ☐ **D** Symptomatic diverticulosis needs treatment with a high fibre diet
    ☐ **E** Acute diverticulitis is a common complication

9. **Regarding colorectal cancer, in a 60-year-old male TWO of the following symptoms/signs require urgent referral**
    ☐ **A** Change in bowel habit, decreasing frequency of defaecation
    ☐ **B** Rectal bleeding with anal symptoms
    ☐ **C** Lower abdominal pain without evidence of intestinal obstruction
    ☐ **D** Hb that is <11g/dl
    ☐ **E** Abdominal mass in the right iliac fossa

SINGLE BEST ANSWER QUESTIONS

1. **In the treatment of duodenal ulcer which ONE of the following is true?**
   - ☐ **A**   A single daily dose of H_2-receptor antagonists is as effective as multiple doses
   - ☐ **B**   Patients with ulcers resistant to H_2-receptor antagonists should have the dose increased
   - ☐ **C**   The recurrence rate is influenced by the choice of initial drugs for treatment
   - ☐ **D**   Patients who fail to respond to treatment with H_2-antagonists after two months should be tested or treated for *Helicobacter pylori*
   - ☐ **E**   Recurrence after successful treatment may be entirely asymptomatic
   - ☐ **F**   Dual therapy is the best form of H. Pylori eradication

2. **Which ONE of the following is least likely to be associated with jaundice?**
   - ☐ **A**   Arsenic
   - ☐ **B**   Methyldopa
   - ☐ **C**   Atenolol
   - ☐ **D**   Chlorpromazine
   - ☐ **E**   Oral contraceptive pill

3. **Select ONE statement. Ultrasound examination of the biliary system**
   - ☐ **A**   is as accurate as oral cholecystography in demonstrating gall bladder calculi
   - ☐ **B**   will demonstrate the cause of bile duct obstruction in only 25% of cases
   - ☐ **C**   cannot diagnose biliary carcinoma
   - ☐ **D**   yields approximately 50% false-negative results in differentiating bile duct obstruction from non-obstructive jaundice
   - ☐ **E**   cannot be performed in the fasting patient

4. **Select ONE statement. Irritable bowel syndrome**
   - ☐ **A**   may follow an episode of infective diarrhoea
   - ☐ **B**   is a diagnosis which can only be safely made following a normal colonoscopy or barium enema
   - ☐ **C**   is commonly found to have been present in early adult life in patients presenting with diverticular disease in middle age
   - ☐ **D**   rarely presents over the age of 60

5. **Which ONE of the following drugs does not cause constipation?**
   - ☐ **A**   Aluminium trisilicate
   - ☐ **B**   Tricyclic antidepressants
   - ☐ **C**   Oral contraceptives
   - ☐ **D**   Cimetidine
   - ☐ **E**   Iron

6. Select ONE of the following items concerning irritable bowel syndrome

☐ **A**   Is more common in women than in men
☐ **B**   Often presents in middle to old age
☐ **C**   Causes abdominal pain made worse by defaecation
☐ **D**   Causes rectal bleeding
☐ **E**   Seldom affects children

7. Which ONE of the following statements concerning diverticular disease is correct?

☐ **A**   Often occurs without symptoms
☐ **B**   Affects the transverse colon more commonly than the sigmoid colon
☐ **C**   Commonly presents with rectal bleeding
☐ **D**   Should not be treated with morphine as it increases muscle spasm
☐ **E**   Usually requires immediate surgery

INFECTIOUS DISEASES/ HAEMATOLOGY/ IMMUNOLOGY/ ALLERGIES/GENETICS

EXTENDED MATCHING QUESTIONS

THEME: CHROMOSOME DISORDERS

A Autosomal Dominant
B Autosomal Recessive
C X-Linked

For each of the following conditions, select the type of chromosome disorder from the list above. Each option may be used once, more than once or not at all.

1. Haemophilia A ☐

2. Familial Hypercholesterolaemia ☐

3. Cystic Fibrosis ☐

4. Red-Green colour blindness ☐

5. Familial Polyposis Coli ☐

THEME: INFECTIVE AGENTS ASSOCIATED WITH TUMOURS

A   Epstein-Barr virus
B   *Helicobacter pylori*
C   Hepatitis B virus
D   Human herpes virus type 8
E   Human papillomavirus
F   Measles virus
G   Parvovirus

For each of the following tumours, select the infective agent associated with the tumour from the list above. Each option may be used once, more than once or not at all.

6. Gastric lymphoma ☐

7. Hepatocellular carcinoma ☐

8. Kaposi's sarcoma ☐

9. Genital warts ☐

10. Squamous cell carcinoma of cervix ☐

MULTIPLE BEST ANSWER QUESTIONS

1. **Which TWO of the following are NOT typical features of Turner's syndrome?**
   - ☐ **A**   XY genotype
   - ☐ **B**   Tall stature
   - ☐ **C**   Streak ovaries
   - ☐ **D**   Cubitus valgus
   - ☐ **E**   Webbed neck

2. **Select TWO of the following. Pertussis immunisation is contraindicated in a child**
   - ☐ **A**   with atopic eczema
   - ☐ **B**   who develops fever of 40°C within 36 hours of 1st dose of the triple vaccine
   - ☐ **C**   whose maternal uncle is an epileptic
   - ☐ **D**   who develops a severe local reaction at the site where the 1st dose of the triple vaccine was administered
   - ☐ **E**   who had hypocalcaemic fits in the neonatal period

3. **Select THREE diseases that are inherited as autosomal dominant**
   - ☐ **A**   Down's syndrome
   - ☐ **B**   Myotonic dystrophy
   - ☐ **C**   Cystic fibrosis
   - ☐ **D**   Adult polycystic kidney disease
   - ☐ **E**   Huntingdon's chorea

4. **Select THREE statements about diarrhoea in a patient with acquired immune deficiency syndrome (AIDS)**
   - ☐ **A**   May be due to infective proctitis in the anoreceptive homosexual
   - ☐ **B**   May be due to cryptosporidium
   - ☐ **C**   Will require colonoscopy to establish diagnosis
   - ☐ **D**   The faeces should be treated with caution as they are heavily laden with human immunodeficiency virus (HIV)
   - ☐ **E**   May be secondary to small bowel parasites

5. **Which TWO of the following are true of infectious hepatitis?**
   - ☐ **A**   Hepatitis C is food/water borne
   - ☐ **B**   Patients are maximally infectious prior to the onset of jaundice
   - ☐ **C**   Vaccine to hepatitis B may reduce the incidence of hepatoma
   - ☐ **D**   Alkaline phosphatase is rarely more than double the upper limit of the reference range
   - ☐ **E**   Hepatitis D is now the commonest blood borne hepatitis in the UK

6. **Which THREE of the following are features of glandular fever?**
- ☐ **A** Abnormal liver function tests
- ☐ **B** Rash
- ☐ **C** Illness lasts about five days
- ☐ **D** Monospot test is invariably positive
- ☐ **E** Gross cervical lymphadenopathy

7. **Which TWO of the following statements about normal iron metabolism are true?**
- ☐ **A** The normal daily requirement for adults is 1–2 mg
- ☐ **B** Haemoglobin accounts for about 25% of total body iron
- ☐ **C** There is no physiological route for iron excretion
- ☐ **D** Iron is more readily absorbed from vegetables than from meat

8. **Pneumococcal immunisation should be given to which TWO groups of patients?**
- ☐ **A** Who are HIV-positive
- ☐ **B** Who are heterozygous for Hb S
- ☐ **C** Who have had a splenectomy
- ☐ **D** Every five years where indicated
- ☐ **E** Prior to travel to countries with high rates of penicillin-resistant pneumococci

9. **Which THREE groups of patients have increased susceptibility to pneumococcal infections?**
- ☐ **A** Hypothyroidism
- ☐ **B** Post-splenectomy
- ☐ **C** Melanomas
- ☐ **D** Multiple myeloma
- ☐ **E** Anaemia
- ☐ **F** Sickle cell disease

SINGLE BEST ANSWER QUESTIONS

1. Select the statement which is NOT true of measles

☐ **A** Account for 15% of deaths from all causes in children under five in developed countries

☐ **B** May cause recurrent pneumothoraces

☐ **C** May cause corneal ulceration

☐ **D** Is more dangerous in overcrowded households

☐ **E** Establishes lifelong immunity after natural infection

2. Which of the following does NOT result in a depressed immune response?

☐ **A** Obesity

☐ **B** Antibiotic treatment

☐ **C** Renal failure

☐ **D** Old age

☐ **E** Infection

3. Which of the following is NOT associated with red blood cell macrocytosis?

☐ **A** Coeliac disease

☐ **B** Ulcerative colitis

☐ **C** Alcoholism

☐ **D** Aplastic anaemia

4. Which of the following statements about HIV antibody test is NOT true?

☐ **A** The interval between seroconversion and exposure to infection is usually no more than 2 months

☐ **B** A seronegative individual can infect other people

☐ **C** The virus is more readily isolated from blood than from other body fluids

☐ **D** A positive antibody test will always be indicative of infection

☐ **E** Detection of antibodies is the cheapest and most accurate of HIV diagnostic procedures

5. Deficiencies of the following food substances are linked with which ONE of the associated haematological conditions?

☐ **A** Iron and megaloblastic anaemia

☐ **B** Cobalamin and haemolytic anaemia

☐ **C** Folic acid and microcytic anaemia

☐ **D** Vitamin C and microcytic anaemia

6. Which of the following statements is NOT true about sickle cell anaemia?

☐ **A** Folate supplements may prevent aplastic crises

☐ **B** Serum iron is low

☐ **C** Aseptic femoral head necrosis may occur

☐ **D** Priapism is a recognised complication

☐ **E** Pneumococcal immunisation is advised

☐ **F** Recurrent haematuria may occur

7. Which ONE of the following is NOT a complication of rheumatoid disease?

☐ **A**   Finger clubbing
☐ **B**   Baker's synovial cysts
☐ **C**   Pleural effusion
☐ **D**   Leg ulcers
☐ **E**   Pernicious anaemia

PAEDIATRICS

EXTENDED MATCHING QUESTIONS

THEME: COMMON DEVELOPMENTAL MILESTONES

A 3 months
B 6 months
C 9 months
D 12 months
E 18 months

For each of the descriptions, select the single most likely age. Each option may be used once, more than once, or not at all.

1. Says 2–3 words with meaning ☐

2. Sits unsupported and may crawl on abdomen ☐

3. Manages a spoon ☐

4. Builds a 3–4 cube tower ☐

5. Sits supported ☐

6. Holds object placed in hand ☐

7. Walks with one hand held ☐

THEME: ABDOMINAL PAIN IN CHILDREN

A Inguinal hernia
B Urinary tract infection
C Sickle cell disease
D Intussusception
E Acute porphyria
F Diabetic ketoacidosis
G Henoch-Schönlein purpura
H Appendicitis
I Abdominal migraine
J Testicular torsion
K Lead poisoning
L Mesenteric adenitis

From the list of descriptions below, select the most likely diagnosis from the list above. Each option may be used once, more than once or not at all.

8. Usually associated with a rash and joint swelling, often with haematuria ☐

9. Is characterised by periodic bouts of screaming, drawing up of the legs and pallor with blood stained mucus passed in nappies ☐

10. Should be considered in a child with abdominal pain and dysuria, with normal urine ☐

11. May cause referred pain to the abdomen in 25% of cases ☐

12. May be associated with preceding upper respiratory tract symptoms ☐

MULTIPLE BEST ANSWER QUESTIONS

1. Select THREE risk factors for Sudden Infant Death Syndrome
- ☐ **A**   Female sex
- ☐ **B**   Supine sleeping position
- ☐ **C**   Young maternal age
- ☐ **D**   Low parity
- ☐ **E**   Winter months
- ☐ **F**   Respiratory symptoms over the previous few days

2. Select THREE statements about breast-feeding
- ☐ **A**   Is protective against gastrointestinal infections
- ☐ **B**   Reduces the risk of insulin dependent diabetes
- ☐ **C**   Is protective against respiratory diseases
- ☐ **D**   Increases the risk of maternal breast cancer
- ☐ **E**   Increases the likelihood of childhood obesity

3. Select THREE statements relating to Down's syndrome
- ☐ **A**   40% of fetuses with trisomy 21 die between 10–14 weeks
- ☐ **B**   Nuchal scanning involves measuring the fat layer in the fetal neck
- ☐ **C**   Follow up from ultrasound gives detection rates of over 60%
- ☐ **D**   Nuchal scanning has a detection rate of over 75%
- ☐ **E**   The triple test has a higher detection rate than nuchal scanning

4. Select THREE factors that are less common in breast-fed babies
- ☐ **A**   Non-accidental injury
- ☐ **B**   Coeliac disease
- ☐ **C**   Eczema
- ☐ **D**   Urinary tract infections
- ☐ **E**   Cot death

5. Select THREE common features of Down's syndrome
- ☐ **A**   Speckled iris (Brushfield's spots)
- ☐ **B**   Normal IQ
- ☐ **C**   Loose skin on nape of neck
- ☐ **D**   Protruding tongue
- ☐ **E**   Spasticity

6. Select THREE statements regarding congenital dislocation of the hip
- ☐ **A**   It is more common in boys than girls
- ☐ **B**   In carrying out Ortolani's test the hips should be abducted to 70°
- ☐ **C**   Is a cause of delayed walking
- ☐ **D**   Treatment is most effective in infants
- ☐ **E**   When picked up late, requires an open reduction operation

7. **People with Down's syndrome are particularly prone to which TWO conditions?**
   - ☐ **A**   Diabetes insipidus
   - ☐ **B**   Hypothyroidism
   - ☐ **C**   Hyperparathyroidism
   - ☐ **D**   Alzheimer's disease
   - ☐ **E**   Addison's disease

8. **Select TWO of the following statements about nocturnal enuresis**
   - ☐ **A**   Most children with nocturnal enuresis are reliably dry during the day
   - ☐ **B**   By the age of 10 years only about 1% of children suffer nocturnal enuresis
   - ☐ **C**   First born children are more prone to nocturnal enuresis than later children
   - ☐ **D**   Urodynamic studies can often help diagnose the cause of nocturnal enuresis
   - ☐ **E**   Tricyclic drugs are effective by reason of their anticholinergic and antidepressant effects

9. **At the age of eight months, a baby can be expected to do which TWO of the following?**
   - ☐ **A**   Roll over from front to back
   - ☐ **B**   Pick up a small bead between thumb and finger
   - ☐ **C**   Sit up with a straight back
   - ☐ **D**   Say up to five words clearly
   - ☐ **E**   Feed itself with a spoon

SINGLE BEST ANSWER QUESTIONS

1. In congenital dislocation of the hip
- ☐ **A** The incidence is 2–3 per 100 births in the UK
- ☐ **B** The incidence for surgical intervention has changed with screening
- ☐ **C** Splinting carries a risk of avascular necrosis of the femoral head

2. Which of the following statements is NOT true about congenital dislocation of the hips?
- ☐ **A** Is more common in males
- ☐ **B** 90% of dislocatable hips will stabilise in first two months of life
- ☐ **C** Is rare in black Afro-Caribbeans
- ☐ **D** Is best diagnosed using ultrasound rather than X-rays
- ☐ **E** The risk is increased if positive family history

3. Which of the following is true of puberty?
- ☐ **A** In normal girls the pubertal growth spurt precedes the menarche
- ☐ **B** The first sign of puberty in the male is development of pubic hair
- ☐ **C** Precocious puberty is more likely to have a sinister underlying cause in a girl than in a boy
- ☐ **D** Delayed pubertal development is most commonly due to a structural defect causing gonadotrophin deficiency
- ☐ **E** Menarche is a late event in puberty

4. Mrs Fisher brings her 4-week-old daughter in to see you, complaining that Britney has terrible colic and she would like something for it. Which one of the following has been shown to be the most effective treatment for infantile colic?
- ☐ **A** Dimethicone
- ☐ **B** Low lactose milk
- ☐ **C** Dicyclomine
- ☐ **D** Carrying the infant during attacks
- ☐ **E** None of the above

PHARMACO-THERAPEUTICS

EXTENDED MATCHING QUESTIONS

THEME: SIMILAR SOUNDING DRUGS

A   Lansoprazole
B   Lofepramine
C   Loperamide
D   Loprazolan
E   Loratidine
F   Lorezepam

For each description below, select the single most likely drug from the above options. Each option may be used once, more than once, or not at all.

1. An antihistamine ☐

2. Can cause abdominal cramps and is used as an adjunct to other treatment in diarrhoea ☐

3. A proton pump inhibitor ☐

4. A hypnotic ☐

5. An anxiolytic and can be used in the treatment of status epilepticus ☐

6. Used in the symptomatic treatment of urticaria ☐

7. Used in the treatment of duodenal ulcers ☐

8. An antidepressant ☐

THEME: SIDE-EFFECTS OF DYSPEPSIA TREATMENT

A Aluminium salts
B H$_2$-receptor antagonists
C Magnesium salts
D Metoclopramide
E Misoprostol
F Omeprazole

For each side-effect, select the single most likely dyspepsia treatment. Each option may be used once, more than once, or not at all.

9. Can cause intermenstrual bleeding ☐

10. Can be associated with postmenopausal bleeding ☐

11. Often causes diarrhoea ☐

12. Can cause severe skin reactions and photosensitivity ☐

13. Frequently causes constipation ☐

14. Is associated with dystonic reactions ☐

15. Can cause galactorrhoea ☐

16. Can cause confusion, which is reversible on stopping the medication ☐

THEME: ANTI-INFECTIVE DRUG SIDE-EFFECTS

A Ciprofloxacin
B Terbinafine
C Zanamivir
D Doxycycline
E Azithromycin
F Metronidazole
G Rifampicin
H Acyclovir

For each side-effect described, select the drug associated with it. Each option may be used once, more than once or not at all.

17. Acute renal failure ☐

18. Bronchospasm ☐

19. Photosensitivity ☐

20. Discoloration of body secretions ☐

21. Tendon damage ☐

22. Disulfiram-like reaction ☐

MULTIPLE BEST ANSWER QUESTIONS

1. **Which TWO of the following drugs should be avoided in renal failure?**
    ☐ **A**   Ampicillin
    ☐ **B**   Oxytetracycline
    ☐ **C**   Aluminium hydroxide
    ☐ **D**   Ferrous sulphate
    ☐ **E**   Nitrofurantoin

2. **Choose TWO of the following statements. Benzodiazepine anxiolytics**
    ☐ **A**   have no active metabolites
    ☐ **B**   differ significantly in their duration of action
    ☐ **C**   differ significantly in their sedative effect relative to anxiolytic activity
    ☐ **D**   increase body sway

3. **Select TWO statements about cannabis**
    ☐ **A**   Is usually smoked but can be ingested or injected intravenously
    ☐ **B**   Usually causes bradycardia
    ☐ **C**   Injections produce severe constipation
    ☐ **D**   Use over many years may impair academic performance, which is reversible on cessation of use
    ☐ **E**   Smoke may be carcinogenic

4. **Aspirin potentiates the therapeutic action of which TWO drugs?**
    ☐ **A**   Warfarin
    ☐ **B**   Probenecid
    ☐ **C**   Indomethacin
    ☐ **D**   Diazepam
    ☐ **E**   Tetracyclines

5. **Which THREE of the following drugs should be avoided or used with caution in renal failure?**
    ☐ **A**   Aspirin
    ☐ **B**   Ampicillin
    ☐ **C**   Glibenclamide
    ☐ **D**   Somatropin
    ☐ **E**   Atorvastatin

6. **Which TWO of the following are associated with cannabis abuse?**
    ☐ **A**   Irreversible reduction in academic performance
    ☐ **B**   Persistent bradycardia
    ☐ **C**   Hypotension
    ☐ **D**   Hypertension
    ☐ **E**   Status epilepticus

7. **THREE recognised side-effects of benzodiazepines are**
- ☐ **A**   confusion
- ☐ **B**   impaired driving skills
- ☐ **C**   potentiation of the effects of alcohol
- ☐ **D**   aplastic anaemia
- ☐ **E**   convulsions

8. **THREE of the following drugs are safe to use in combination with warfarin**
- ☐ **A**   Ranitidine
- ☐ **B**   Co-trimoxazole
- ☐ **C**   Carbamazepine
- ☐ **D**   Ibuprofen
- ☐ **E**   Salbutamol

9. **Which TWO of the following drugs are suitable for breast-feeding women?**
- ☐ **A**   Sulphonamides
- ☐ **B**   Aspirin
- ☐ **C**   Lithium
- ☐ **D**   Cephalosporins
- ☐ **E**   Tricyclic antidepressants

10. **There is reduced effectiveness of the combined oral contraceptive pill following interaction with which THREE of the following?**
- ☐ **A**   Rifamycin
- ☐ **B**   Carbamazepine
- ☐ **C**   Warfarin
- ☐ **D**   Lisinopril
- ☐ **E**   Griseofulvin

11. **Which THREE of the following drugs can be safely used in pregnancy with medical advice?**
- ☐ **A**   Piperazine
- ☐ **B**   Simvastatin
- ☐ **C**   Enalapril
- ☐ **D**   Chlorpheniramine
- ☐ **E**   Paracetamol

12. **Which TWO of the following side-effects are linked with non-steroidal anti-inflammatory drugs?**
- ☐ **A**   Hypokalaemia
- ☐ **B**   Polycythaemia
- ☐ **C**   Neutrophilia
- ☐ **D**   Thrombocytopenia
- ☐ **E**   Hypocalcaemia

SINGLE BEST ANSWER QUESTIONS

1. Which ONE of the following drugs is contraindicated in breast-feeding?
- ☐ **A** Warfarin
- ☐ **B** Senna
- ☐ **C** Digoxin
- ☐ **D** Paracetamol
- ☐ **E** Cimetidine

2. Which ONE of these statements about Zanamivir (Relenza) is NOT correct?
- ☐ **A** Inhibits viral replication
- ☐ **B** Does not work with Influenza B infections
- ☐ **C** Is given as a nasal spray or dry powder inhaler
- ☐ **D** Is of particular benefit when symptoms have been present less than 30 hours
- ☐ **E** May exacerbate asthma
- ☐ **F** Enables patients to return to work more quickly

3. Which ONE of these statements about St John's wort is NOT true?
- ☐ **A** Is no more effective than placebo in depression
- ☐ **B** Can induce liver enzymes
- ☐ **C** Is used widely in the UK
- ☐ **D** Interacts with digoxin
- ☐ **E** Interacts with warfarin

4. Which ONE of the following is NOT a toxic effect of digoxin therapy?
- ☐ **A** Abdominal pain
- ☐ **B** Visual disturbance
- ☐ **C** T wave inversion
- ☐ **D** Prolonged PR interval
- ☐ **E** Anorexia

5. Which ONE of the following statements is NOT true about Warfarin?
- ☐ **A** Reduces vitamin K dependent clotting factors
- ☐ **B** Reacts with ampicillin to increase anticoagulant effect
- ☐ **C** Appears in breast milk in quantities too small to affect the baby
- ☐ **D** Has an increased anticoagulant effect with griseofulvin therapy

6. Which ONE of the following is true about Glibenclamide?
- ☐ **A** Has a shorter half-life than chlorpropamide
- ☐ **B** Does not cross the placenta
- ☐ **C** Is safe in renal impairment
- ☐ **D** Is safe to use in the elderly

PSYCHIATRY/ NEUROLOGY

EXTENDED MATCHING QUESTIONS

THEME: SECTIONS OF THE MENTAL HEALTH ACT

A   Section 2
B   Section 3
C   Section 4
D   Section 5
E   Section 7

For each of the statements, select the single most likely option. Each of the options may be used once, more than once, or not at all.

1. Is suitable to use when considering guardianship   ☐

2. Is most suitable for a patient with a recurrence of a mental illness associated with non-compliance with treatment   ☐

3. Is used in an emergency to bring someone into hospital for a full assessment of the mental state   ☐

4. Is used in an emergency to keep someone in hospital pending a further assessment   ☐

5. Is normally used to admit a patient to hospital for a full assessment of the mental state   ☐

THEME: HEADACHES

A Cluster headaches
B Migraine
C Referred from neck
D Tension headaches

For each of the descriptions, select the most likely type of headache. Each option may be used once, more than once, or not at all.

6. The patient will commonly show pallor ☐

7. The pain is typically diffuse or bilateral ☐

8. The pain is described as a weight on the top of the head or as a band ☐

9. The patient often experiences flushing ☐

10. The patient often complains of a watery eye ☐

THEME: DISC LESIONS

A At L2–L3 level
B At L5–S1 level
C Central disc prolapse

For each of the descriptions, select the most likely level of disc lesion. Each option may be used, once, more than once, or not at all.

11. There will be characteristically loss of ankle reflex ☐

12. There will usually be loss of bladder function ☐

13. The femoral stretch test will be positive ☐

THEME: QUESTIONNAIRES

A CAGE
B MAST
C CRATE
D EAT
E SCOFF

For each of the descriptions, select the single most likely questionnaire. Each option may be used once, more than once, or not at all.

14. This is a questionnaire to find people with alcohol problems, who commonly score over 6 with these questions ☐

15. This looks at people with eating disorders ☐

16. This looks for people with alcohol problems who will probably score between 2 and 4 ☐

17. This questionnaire asks, among other questions, whether the person has been arrested for drunken driving ☐

THEME: HEADACHE

A   Cluster headache
B   Tension headache
C   Temporal arteritis
D   Migraine with aura
E   Subarachnoid haemorrhage
F   Sinusitis
G   Migraine without aura
H   Chronic daily headache
I   Coital cephalgia
J   Trigeminal neuralgia

For each of the descriptions listed below, select the single most appropriate answer. Each answer may be used once, more than once or not at all.

18. May occur every day, be continuous and worsen through the day. Rarely disturb sleep; patients can usually work through them. Often band-like with associated neck and shoulder stiffness.

19. Seen mostly in men, a sudden onset of severe pain. May be confused with subarachnoid haemorrhage.

20. Characterised by bouts of daily pain occurring for weeks or months at a time, always unilateral and centered on the eye or cheek, often with lacrimation

21. Causes recurrent severe unilateral headache with nausea and photophobia, often preceded by a prodromal phase

22. May rapidly cause blindness if untreated

23. Is a contraindication to the combined contraceptive pill

THEME: PSYCHIATRIC COMPLAINTS

A   Obsessive-compulsive personality disorder
B   Schizoid personality disorder
C   Borderline personality disorder
D   Conversion disorder
E   Post traumatic stress disorder
F   Drug-induced psychosis
G   Bipolar disorder
H   Schizophrenia
I   Dementia
J   Anxiety disorder

For each clinical scenario described below, select the single most likely diagnosis from the list above. Each answer may be used once, more than once or not at all.

24. A 77-year-old man complains that he cannot play bridge any more due to his inability to memorise hands. Despite his legendary recall of people long since passed, his wife says they frequently argue about his failure to remember what they need from the shops.

25. A 44-year-old woman is brought in by her estranged partner having awoken that morning unable to speak. He is very concerned but she is able to put a brave face on things. She can cough and swallow and ENT examination is normal.

26. Mrs Smith, a 33-year-old woman, was involved in a minor road traffic accident last year. She frequently suffers a dry mouth, difficulty breathing and palpitations. She has trouble sleeping and her memory has deteriorated.

27. A 22-year-old man asks for a sick note to cover his absence from community service last week. He has been in prison for joyriding and theft, and on occasions has threatened suicide. The receptionists in the past have complained about his aggressive and intimidating behaviour.

28. You are called by a neighbour to visit a 67-year-old woman with a previous history of depression. He found her dancing in the garden naked at 3 am last night. She has not slept for days and is bizarrely dressed. She denies there is a problem; she feels fantastic.

29. Since starting university Tom has become interested in the paranormal, is increasingly dishevelled and has been seen talking to himself. His mother says he recently covered the TV screen with paper. He is suspicious and his speech seems to flit from one unrelated theme to another.

THEME: MIGRAINE

A   IM Pethidine
B   Aspirin
C   PR diclofenac
D   Cocodamol
E   Sumatriptan
F   Avoidance of trigger factors
G   Referral to neurology outpatients
H   Emergency medical referral
I   Ergotamine

For each of the descriptions below, select the most appropriate option from the list above. Each option may be used once, more than once or not at all.

30. First-line treatment ☐

31. Should be considered as a prophylactic measure in all patients ☐

32. Should be considered if first-line treatment fails to abort an attack ☐

33. For regular severe attacks, unresponsive to simple remedies, should be taken as soon as possible after an attack starts ☐

34. Is a contraindication to combined oral contraceptive use ☐

35. Should be considered for sudden onset severe headaches with atypical features ☐

THEME: HEADACHES

A Alcoholism
B Brain tumour
C Carbon monoxide poisoning
D Cervical spondylosis
E Depression
F Migraine
G Temporal arteritis
H Tension headache

Select the most likely diagnosis as the cause of the headache. Each option may be used once, more than once, or not at all.

36. A 70-year-old man with a three week history of left-sided headache and one day of blurring vision ☐

37. A 20-year-old girl recently moved in with her boyfriend, complaining of recent onset of frequent headaches, usually on the right-side, accompanied by nausea ☐

38. A 55-year-old male General Practitioner with morning headaches over the last six months, accompanied by strange avoidance behaviour, vomiting and weight loss ☐

39. A 35-year-old lady with polyarthralgia, muscle pains, palpitations and lethargy ☐

40. A 25-year-old who has just moved into your area into a bedsit, who calls you out with headache, vomiting and says she is unable to get out of bed, but who looks remarkably well in colour ☐

THEME: MRC SCALE FOR MUSCLE POWER

A 0
B ½
C 1
D 2
E 3
F 4
G 4½
H 5

For each of the descriptions, select the most likely number. Each of the options may be used once, more than once, or not at all.

41. Movement overcomes gravity plus added resistance ☐

42. No movement of joint, but visible muscle contraction ☐

43. Normal power ☐

THEME: NERVE ROOT LESIONS

A   C4
B   C5
C   C6
D   C6/7
E   L3/4
F   L5/S1
G   S1/S2

For each of the clinical scenarios, select the single most appropriate nerve root lesion. Each option may be used once, more than once, or not at all.

44. Absent ankle reflex and poor foot plantar flexion, but knee flexion intact. ☐

45. Absent biceps reflex and poor shoulder abduction. ☐

46. Absent supinator reflex and poor elbow flexion, but triceps reflex present. ☐

47. Absent knee reflex and poor knee extension and foot dorsiflexion. ☐

MULTIPLE BEST ANSWER QUESTIONS

1. **In a 70-year-old man with tremor of the upper limbs, essential tremor rather than Parkinson's disease is more likely to be the cause in which TWO of the following?**
    ☐ **A** The tremor is worst at rest
    ☐ **B** The tremor is relieved with alcohol
    ☐ **C** The tremor is exacerbated by anxiety
    ☐ **D** The tremor is predominantly postural
    ☐ **E** There is rigidity

2. **Select FOUR important risk factors for suicide**
    ☐ **A** Recent self harm
    ☐ **B** Female
    ☐ **C** Married
    ☐ **D** Unemployed
    ☐ **E** Severity of depression
    ☐ **F** Active plans
    ☐ **G** Passive thoughts about being harmed

3. **Select THREE factors which predispose to major depression**
    ☐ **A** A professional background
    ☐ **B** A first degree relative with major depression
    ☐ **C** The presence of more than three children in the house
    ☐ **D** Employment in the same company for more than 10 years
    ☐ **E** Loss of a parent before 11 years of age

4. **Select TWO of the following statements regarding compensation neurosis**
    ☐ **A** It has a recognised association with major rather than minor accidents
    ☐ **B** It occurs particularly after head injuries sustained at work
    ☐ **C** Settlement of a compensation claim is followed by improvement in patients with severe symptoms
    ☐ **D** Malingering accounts for at least 30% of cases
    ☐ **E** Irritability is a recognised feature

5. **Select THREE statements about agoraphobia**
    ☐ **A** Usually starts before puberty
    ☐ **B** Occurs more often in women than men
    ☐ **C** Can be effectively treated by systematic desensitisation
    ☐ **D** Becomes worse during periods of depression
    ☐ **E** Can usually be traced back to traumatic events in childhood

6. Select THREE of the following statements concerning grief reaction
- ☐ **A** Is typically self-limiting
- ☐ **B** Characteristically includes denial
- ☐ **C** Is best treated with tricyclic antidepressants
- ☐ **D** Typically includes suicidal ideas
- ☐ **E** Is a form of psychosis

7. Select TWO of the following statements about anxiety states
- ☐ **A** Chest pain may be a presenting symptom
- ☐ **B** May present with persistent memory impairment
- ☐ **C** Difficulty in exhaling is common
- ☐ **D** Low mood and early morning wakening are invariably present
- ☐ **E** Sweating is quite common

8. Select TWO of the following about obsessive-compulsive disorder
- ☐ **A** Obsessional thoughts are recognised by patients as being their own
- ☐ **B** Women are more commonly affected than men
- ☐ **C** Obsessional thoughts are usually pleasant in nature
- ☐ **D** Depression is unusual
- ☐ **E** Two-thirds of cases have improved at the end of one year

9. Select THREE Schneiderian first rank symptoms of schizophrenia
- ☐ **A** Thought insertion
- ☐ **B** Visual hallucinations
- ☐ **C** Suicidal ideas
- ☐ **D** Passivity phenomena
- ☐ **E** Thought broadcast

10. Select THREE of the following. An acute confusional state is
- ☐ **A** often responsive to tricyclic antidepressant drug therapy
- ☐ **B** a characteristic feature of myxoedema
- ☐ **C** characterised by loss of memory for recent events
- ☐ **D** typically reversible
- ☐ **E** more common with pre-existing brain disease

11. Select THREE characteristic features of hypomania
- ☐ **A** Flight of ideas
- ☐ **B** Thought insertion
- ☐ **C** Sexual promiscuity
- ☐ **D** Delusions of bodily illness
- ☐ **E** Sleep disturbance

12. Select THREE typical features of alcohol withdrawal
- [ ] **A**   Dehydration
- [ ] **B**   Visual hallucinations
- [ ] **C**   Passivity feelings
- [ ] **D**   Tremor
- [ ] **E**   Confabulation

13. Select TWO features of hysteria
- [ ] **A**   The physical symptom is produced deliberately
- [ ] **B**   It may be associated with a depressive illness
- [ ] **C**   It is associated with 'la belle indifference'
- [ ] **D**   It characteristically occurs for the first time in middle age
- [ ] **E**   The physical symptoms and signs closely resemble those of organic disease

14. Select FOUR of the following statements about suicide
- [ ] **A**   Two-thirds of these who die by suicide have told someone of their intention
- [ ] **B**   Asking about suicidal intent will increase the risk of suicide
- [ ] **C**   Patients with chronic physical illness are at decreased risk
- [ ] **D**   It is associated with alcohol abuse
- [ ] **E**   It is most common in young women
- [ ] **F**   Patients recently bereaved are at increased risk
- [ ] **G**   Unemployed patients are at more risk than those in stressful jobs

15. Select TWO good prognostic signs of schizophrenia
- [ ] **A**   Early onset
- [ ] **B**   Depressive features
- [ ] **C**   Echolalia
- [ ] **D**   Preservation of affect
- [ ] **E**   Visual hallucinations

16. Select TWO of the following statements. Multiple sclerosis
- [ ] **A**   has a higher prevalence in tropical zones than in temperate zones
- [ ] **B**   presents as a single symptom in most patients
- [ ] **C**   may present with diplopia due to optic nerve involvement
- [ ] **D**   does not cause progressive disability in up to one third of patients
- [ ] **E**   very rarely causes sensory disturbance of the limbs

17. Select THREE symptoms which are commonly associated with Bell's palsy
- [ ] **A**   Dry eye
- [ ] **B**   Hyperacusis
- [ ] **C**   Dry mouth
- [ ] **D**   Loss of taste
- [ ] **E**   Postauricular pain

18. Select THREE of the following statements. In the leg

☐ **A** spasticity in a patient with hemiplegia is most pronounced in the extensor muscles

☐ **B** weakness in a patient with hemiplegia is most pronounced in the flexor muscles

☐ **C** sensory loss affecting skin over the lateral aspect of the lower leg may be due to a femoral nerve palsy

☐ **D** weakness of knee extension may be due to a sciatic nerve palsy

☐ **E** foot drop may be due to a common peroneal nerve palsy

19. Select TWO statements about multiple sclerosis

☐ **A** Onset after the age of 40 years indicates a better prognosis

☐ **B** Magnetic resonance imaging may be useful in confirming the diagnosis

☐ **C** Initial presentation with motor symptoms indicates a better prognosis

☐ **D** A homonymous hemianopia is a common feature

☐ **E** Red-green colour vision may be impaired

20. Select TWO comments about stroke

☐ **A** The third most common cause of death in the UK

☐ **B** More commonly caused by infarction than haemorrhage

☐ **C** More common among people from higher socio-economic classes

☐ **D** More likely to be fatal if caused by infarction than haemorrhage

☐ **E** Linked to raised systolic blood pressure but not diastolic

SINGLE BEST ANSWER QUESTIONS

1. Which ONE of the following is true of Alzheimer's disease?
- [ ] **A** Behavioural disturbance is an early clinical manifestation
- [ ] **B** Extensor plantar responses and myoclonus are early clinical features
- [ ] **C** The EEG is usually normal
- [ ] **D** It is associated with a predominantly frontal cortical distribution of pathology
- [ ] **E** It is usually familial
- [ ] **F** It is the commonest cause of dementia

2. In the differential diagnosis of dementia which ONE of the following is true?
- [ ] **A** A multi-infarct aetiology is more common than the Alzheimer's type
- [ ] **B** A CT scan will reliably distinguish between Alzheimer's and multi-infarct dementia
- [ ] **C** In Alzheimer's disease a gait disorder is seen at an early stage
- [ ] **D** In Creutzfeldt-Jakob disease an EEG may be characteristic

3. Which ONE of the following is true with regard to alcohol?
- [ ] **A** Consumption of 7–21 units per month is associated with the lowest mortality
- [ ] **B** Problems can almost all be identified by a raised MCV and raised gamma GT
- [ ] **C** Problems may be picked up by the use of a CAGE questionnaire, with only 25% of those with problems scoring 2 or more

4. Which ONE of the following factors does not indicate an increased risk of suicide in a depressed patient?
- [ ] **A** A direct statement of intent to commit suicide
- [ ] **B** Hopelessness
- [ ] **C** Pressure of serious physical illness
- [ ] **D** Living alone
- [ ] **E** Presence of paranoid delusions

5. Which ONE of the following is NOT true of chronic fatigue syndrome?
- [ ] **A** Previous psychiatric illness is a recognised risk factor
- [ ] **B** A mild rise in creatine phosphokinase is commonly detected
- [ ] **C** Persistent viral antigen is detected in a minority of patients
- [ ] **D** Decreased physical activity is a risk factor for the continuation of fatigue
- [ ] **E** The majority of affected patients fulfil psychiatric criteria for depression

6. **When starting a course of tricyclic antidepressants, which ONE piece of advice from the following information may reasonably be given to patients?**
   - ☐ **A** They should expect the drug to take effect within 24 hours
   - ☐ **B** They should avoid cheese
   - ☐ **C** They may experience a dry mouth at first
   - ☐ **D** Their skin may become sensitive to sunlight
   - ☐ **E** It may help them to lose weight

7. **Which ONE of the following statements regarding tricyclic antidepressants is false?**
   - ☐ **A** Are contraindicated in patients with glaucoma
   - ☐ **B** May cause a dry mouth
   - ☐ **C** Are safe in patients anticoagulated with warfarin
   - ☐ **D** Are contraindicated in patients with ischaemic heart disease
   - ☐ **E** Can cause a fine tremor and unco-ordination

8. **You see a 71-year-old man who 8 days ago experienced an attack of shingles. He now complains of persistent pain. You make a diagnosis of post-herpetic neuralgia. Which ONE of the following is the single best treatment?**
   - ☐ **A** Acyclovir
   - ☐ **B** Topical hydrocortisone
   - ☐ **C** Topical capsaicin
   - ☐ **D** Oral gabapentin
   - ☐ **E** Epidural morphine

9. **Which ONE of these structures is NOT involved in motor neurone disease?**
   - ☐ **A** Posterior horns of the spinal cord
   - ☐ **B** Corticospinal tract
   - ☐ **C** Corticobulbar fibres originating in the motor and pre-motor cortex
   - ☐ **D** Nuclei of the nerves to the bulbar musculature
   - ☐ **E** Anterior horns of the spinal cord

10. **Which ONE of the following treatments may reduce the severity of relapse in multiple sclerosis (MS)?**
   - ☐ **A** Pulsed high dose methylprednisolone
   - ☐ **B** Adrenocortical trophic hormone (ACTH)
   - ☐ **C** Hyperbaric oxygen
   - ☐ **D** Azathioprine
   - ☐ **E** Linoleic acid supplementation

11. Which ONE of the following statements about migraine is true?

- ☐ **A**   Over half of all patients have their first attack before the age of 20
- ☐ **B**   Over half of all patients have an aura before the headache
- ☐ **C**   Frequency of attacks may vary from occasional to daily
- ☐ **D**   To make the diagnosis of migraine the headache must be unilateral
- ☐ **E**   Vasoconstriction of cerebral blood vessels is characteristic of migraine

12. You see a 42-year-old man with backache. Which ONE of the following symptoms may indicate potentially serious pathology and hence require further investigation or referral if the symptoms do not resolve?

- ☐ **A**   Unilateral leg pain worse than low back pain
- ☐ **B**   Pain radiating to the buttocks
- ☐ **C**   Perineal anaesthesia
- ☐ **D**   Presentation under 20 years or over 55 years at initial presentation
- ☐ **E**   Localised neurological signs

REPRODUCTIVE/ RENAL

EXTENDED MATCHING QUESTIONS

THEME: COMMON CANCERS

A Breast cancer
B Cervical cancer
C Endometrial cancer
D Ovarian cancer

For each of the descriptions, select the single most likely cancer. Each of the options may be used once, more than once, or not at all.

1. The most common malignant tumour that affects women only. ☐

2. Associated with an early menarche, rapid establishment of regular menstruation, obesity and high alcohol intake. ☐

3. Linked with unopposed oestrogen use; progestogen oral contraception may be protective. ☐

4. More common in nulliparous and subfertile women, and sometimes has a familial tendency. ☐

5. Linked with early teenage sexual intercourse, increased parity and smoking. ☐

6. Is usually a squamous carcinoma linked to oral contraceptive use of more than 10 years. ☐

THEME: MENSTRUAL DISTURBANCES

A Fibroids
B Pelvic inflammatory disease
C Cervical erosion
D Normal menstrual cycle
E Endometriosis
F Climacteric
G Menorrhagia
H Polycystic ovary syndrome
I Breakthrough bleeding

For each patient with menstrual symptoms below, select the single most likely diagnosis. Each option may be used once, more than once or not at all.

7. A 24-year-old woman with no previous gynaecological history of note complains of increased clear, non-offensive vaginal discharge and occasional post-coital spotting since restarting the pill after her last pregnancy. She is otherwise asymptomatic.

8. A 46-year-old woman complains that over the last 18 months her periods have been increasingly irregular, with intervals ranging from 1 week to 6 weeks between bleeds. Four months ago she was found to have a mild iron deficient anaemia and tells you that on occasion she floods.

9. A 37-year-old Nigerian lady complains of heavy periods, urinary frequency and a progressive abdominal distension.

10. A 36-year-old complains of a long history of dysmenorrhoea, deep dyspareunia and menorrhagia. She has come requesting referral for infertility.

11. Miss Smith, a 22-year-old student consults you about her irregular cycles, which she says have been irregular for several years. Review of her records show she has been seen in the past for dietary advice and has had Dianette for acne. She is not currently taking any medications.

12. A 22-year-old nurse complains that since stopping the pill, her periods have been irregular, usually 2–3 days early each month.

THEME: CONTRACEPTION

A   Combined pill
B   Minipill
C   Levonelle-2
D   IUD insertion
E   Diaphragm
F   Triphasic pill
G   Implanon
H   Mirena IUS
I   Depo-Provera
J   Norplant
K   Sterilisation
L   HRT

For each of the situations described below, select the most appropriate choice from the list above. Each answer may be used once, more than once or not at all.

13. A 41-year-old woman attends for a routine pill check. She is on Microgynon. Review of her notes show she has in the past tried barrier methods and fallen pregnant. She hates the thought of the coil. She is obese. Her blood pressure is 160/100 but she tells you that '…she has just run up the hill.' ☐

14. Miss Jones is leaving next week to spend nine months travelling around the world in her gap year. She does not have a boyfriend but would like something just in case. She is concerned about the risk of DVT. ☐

15. Late on Friday afternoon a 27-year-old mother of two comes to see you in surgery asking for contraception. After appropriate counselling you give her a prescription for Microgynon 30 to start at her next period. The following Tuesday she telephones you to say that she had intercourse on Friday night and would like the 'Morning after Pill'. ☐

16. An 18-year-old student wants to go on the pill. Review of her previous medical history shows she has in the past had migraines associated with numbness in her arms, although these are now controlled with ergotamine, although she often forgets to take it. ☐

17. At the well woman clinic you see a woman who has not had a period for five months; blood tests have shown that she is perimenopausal. She is in a stable sexual relationship and wants contraception but does not like the idea of the pill. ☐

18. You see a 42-year-old woman who has suffered menorrhagia with flooding increasingly over the last two years. She has had minimal benefit from tranexamic acid but doesn't want a hysterectomy. She is currently on the combined pill. ☐

MULTIPLE BEST ANSWER QUESTIONS

1. **Choose TWO of the following statements regarding postnatal depression**
   - ☐ **A** Can be treated with hormonal therapy
   - ☐ **B** Affects over 10% of deliveries
   - ☐ **C** Rarely becomes chronic or recurrent
   - ☐ **D** Is frequently undetected
   - ☐ **E** Has no relationship to previous psychiatric history

2. **Select TWO of these statements about postnatal depression**
   - ☐ **A** Occurs in up to 25% of women after giving birth
   - ☐ **B** Is more common in women with a history of psychiatric illness
   - ☐ **C** Is more common in women who have had obstetric complications
   - ☐ **D** Results in suicide attempts by up to 10% of affected women
   - ☐ **E** In breast-feeding mothers cannot be treated by antidepressant drugs because they are secreted into the breast milk in large amounts

3. **Which THREE of the following statements about breast-feeding are true?**
   - ☐ **A** Foremilk contains more fat than hindmilk
   - ☐ **B** Human milk is low in protein compared with cows' milk
   - ☐ **C** Cows' milk and human milk have similar fat contents
   - ☐ **D** Vitamin K levels are low in breast milk
   - ☐ **E** An exclusively breast-fed baby's iron stores become low one month after birth

4. **Choose TWO of the following statements. Hormone Replacement Therapy in the majority of menopausal women**
   - ☐ **A** would reduce hot flushes and night sweats
   - ☐ **B** improves libido
   - ☐ **C** reduces the risk of osteoporosis
   - ☐ **D** causes weight gain
   - ☐ **E** increases the risk of breast cancer

5. **Select TWO of these items. Chlamydia infections**
   - ☐ **A** are asymptomatic in 25% of cases
   - ☐ **B** do not usually affect subsequent fertility
   - ☐ **C** can be tested for with urine samples
   - ☐ **D** are the commonest curable STD in the developed world
   - ☐ **E** are found in about 10% of the population

6. **Select TWO statements about carcinoma of the cervix**
   - ☐ **A** Majority of women with this have HPV infection
   - ☐ **B** Vast majority of women with HPV do not develop this
   - ☐ **C** Death rate is increasing

7. **Select FOUR of the following items. Contraception using the combined oral contraceptive pill**

☐ **A**   suppresses benign breast disease
☐ **B**   suppresses ovarian cysts
☐ **C**   decreases pelvic inflammatory disease
☐ **D**   decreases incidence of ovarian cancer
☐ **E**   decreases the risk of arterial disease
☐ **F**   decreases the rate of breast cancer

8. **Select THREE of the following items concerning hormone replacement therapy**

☐ **A**   Has been extensively studied in random controlled trials with placebo comparison
☐ **B**   Controls symptoms of peri-menopausal depression
☐ **C**   Prevents osteoporosis
☐ **D**   Can cause deep venous thrombosis
☐ **E**   Use is associated with a longer life

9. **Select TWO statements concerning hormonal post-coital contraception**

☐ **A**   Must be used within 48 hours of unprotected sex
☐ **B**   Involves two doses spaced 12 hours apart
☐ **C**   Invariably contains oestrogens and progestogens
☐ **D**   Should be repeated 72 hours later if vomiting occurs
☐ **E**   Should be followed up if there is a delay of the next expected menstrual cycle

10. **Antenatal women should be advised about which THREE of the following?**

☐ **A**   Take folic acid supplements for the first trimester
☐ **B**   Take vitamin supplements, in particular vitamin A, for the first trimester
☐ **C**   Take iron supplements throughout the pregnancy if iron deficient
☐ **D**   Avoid all cheeses
☐ **E**   Avoid all pates

11. **THREE recognised causes of menorrhagia are**

☐ **A**   Thyrotoxicosis
☐ **B**   Fibroids
☐ **C**   Intra-uterine contraceptive device
☐ **D**   Pelvic inflammatory disease
☐ **E**   Anorexia

12. **THREE of the following factors pre-dispose to pre-eclampsia**

☐ **A**   Diabetes
☐ **B**   Multiparous women
☐ **C**   Twin pregnancies
☐ **D**   Hydatidiform mole
☐ **E**   Myxoedema

13. **Regarding contraception counselling for patients under 16, select TWO statements**
- [ ] **A** They should always be accompanied by an adult
- [ ] **B** A full sexual history is not always essential
- [ ] **C** The combined oral contraceptive pill is often the most appropriate form of contraception
- [ ] **D** IUCD can be inserted in a nulliparous patient
- [ ] **E** Mirena is an option

14. **Select THREE items which are true in relation to puerperal psychosis**
- [ ] **A** is much more frequent in primiparous women
- [ ] **B** usually begins in the first two weeks after delivery
- [ ] **C** recurrence in subsequent pregnancies is the rule
- [ ] **D** usually has an insidious onset
- [ ] **E** normally has a good prognosis
- [ ] **F** is the most common presentation in a depressive illness

15. **Choose TWO statements regarding perimenopausal contraception**
- [ ] **A** FSH levels are reliable in women using the combined oral contraception pill
- [ ] **B** FSH levels are reliable in woman using the progesterone only pill
- [ ] **C** A copper containing IUD inserted at age 40 needs changing every three years
- [ ] **D** Mirena is a possible form of contraception

16. **Select THREE statements. Puerperal psychosis**
- [ ] **A** usually begins within two days after childbirth
- [ ] **B** is commonly accompanied by clouding of consciousness
- [ ] **C** has a favourable prognosis
- [ ] **D** characteristically includes auditory hallucinations
- [ ] **E** characteristically includes obsessional ruminations

17. **Choose THREE statements about torsion of the testis**
- [ ] **A** Is most common in teenagers
- [ ] **B** Usually presents with abdominal pain and vomiting after trauma
- [ ] **C** Does not always require urgent referral
- [ ] **D** Non-viable testis should always be removed
- [ ] **E** An average General Practitioner is never likely to come across the condition

18. **Select TWO items regarding benign prostatic hypertrophy**
- [ ] **A** Is increasing in prevalence
- [ ] **B** Nocturia is a good diagnostic feature of the condition
- [ ] **C** Beta-blockers are drugs of choice in managing mild conditions
- [ ] **D** The number of transurethral prostectomy operations is increasing in the UK
- [ ] **E** It is essential to do a PSA test once the condition is diagnosed

19. Select TWO of these statement concerning prostatic cancer

☐ **A**   Is seldom seen in men under the age of 50

☐ **B**   Is usually a poorly differentiated cancer

☐ **C**   Can be accurately diagnosed using prostate-specific antigen

☐ **D**   Can be treated by radiotherapy in the early stages as effectively as by surgery

☐ **E**   Responds objectively in almost all cases to hormone therapy

SINGLE BEST ANSWER QUESTIONS

1. **Which ONE of the following is NOT true about childhood urinary tract infection?**
   - ☐ A   Has a benign outcome in most children
   - ☐ B   Is diagnosed once culture of fresh urine yields pure bacterial growth of greater than 10^5/ml
   - ☐ C   Is associated with vesico-ureteric reflux in 2 out of 3 affected children
   - ☐ D   Is caused by an unsuspected surgical disorder in 5% of children
   - ☐ E   Should be treated by combination antimicrobial therapy

2. **Which ONE of the following is true with regard to breast cancer?**
   - ☐ A   Is the second most common cancer in women
   - ☐ B   Incidence equates to a 1:25 lifetime risk for each woman
   - ☐ C   Survival is improved by 15–20% by Tamoxifen with oestrogen receptor positive tumours
   - ☐ D   Treatment with tamoxifen has no effect on the risk of a further cancer in the other breast
   - ☐ E   Screening with short intervals between screening episodes would prevent more deaths

3. **Taking oral contraceptive steroids makes a woman more susceptible to which ONE of the following?**
   - ☐ A   Benign breast disease
   - ☐ B   Carcinoma of the ovary
   - ☐ C   Venous thrombosis
   - ☐ D   Carcinoma of the uterus
   - ☐ E   Pancreatitis

4. **Which ONE of the following is true of endometrial cancer?**
   - ☐ A   It is more common among women using progestogen containing oral contraceptives
   - ☐ B   It is usually poorly differentiated
   - ☐ C   It is now most effectively treated by a combination of radiotherapy and hormone-based chemotherapy
   - ☐ D   It is characterised by late blood borne metastasis, usually to the lung
   - ☐ E   It has usually spread to local lymph glands at diagnosis

5. **ONE medical factor considered in the use of the oral contraceptive pill is**
   - ☐ A   Progesterone only preparations increase the blood pressure
   - ☐ B   A previous history of arterial or venous thrombosis is a contraindication for a progesterone only pill
   - ☐ C   Combined preparations should be avoided in patients with sickle cell disease
   - ☐ D   Malignant melanomas may be oestrogen dependent
   - ☐ E   The progesterone only pill is preferred in patients with epilepsy

6. Which ONE of the following statements best describes bladder cancer?

☐ A   Bladder cancer is usually a squamous carcinoma

☐ B   At presentation, most tumours have invaded the muscle of the bladder wall

☐ C   Survival correlates well with TNM staging at presentation

☐ D   Superficial tumours, if effectively treated by endoscopic resection and diathermy, seldom become invasive

☐ E   Chemotherapy for metastatic disease is ineffective and seldom used

7. Which ONE statement is true for prostate cancer?

☐ A   Is the second commonest cancer in men

☐ B   Is the commonest cause of cancer death in men

☐ C   Already has secondary spread in 10% at diagnosis in UK

☐ D   Terminal events do not usually involve pain

☐ E   Screening does not appear to increase survival

RESPIRATORY MEDICINE

EXTENDED MATCHING QUESTIONS

THEME: BREATHLESSNESS

A   Allergic alveolitis
B   Asthma
C   Hay fever
D   Lung cancer
E   Myocardial infarction
F   Pulmonary embolism

For each patient with breathlessness, select the single most likely diagnosis. Each option can be used once, more than once or not at all.

1. A 35-year-old non-smoking male, presents with a one month history of breathlessness on exertion, especially in the mornings, productive cough, fever and weight loss of seven pounds. He also complains of pains in his left leg following a fall in his aviary. Occasional crepitations were noted in the chest and his peak flow rate was 650 l/min. The left leg was not swollen but slightly tender over the calf. A chest X-ray showed fine nodulations. ☐

2. A 49-year-old female smoker presents with a short history of cough, haemoptysis and weight loss of five pounds. Peak flow was decreased but clinically chest was clear. Chest X-ray showed opacity near the hilum. ☐

3. A 34-year-old male smoker presents with sore eyes, coryza, sneezing and breathlessness. His chest sounded wheezy and his recorded peak flow was 50% of that predicted for his age and height. Chest X-ray showed hyper-inflated lungs. ☐

4. A 34-year-old female smoker on the combined oral contraceptive pill presents with sudden onset of breathlessness and pain on the left side of the chest. On examination she is sweating profusely, in pain and tachypnoeic. BP was normal. ☐

5. A 59-year-old male smoker present with sudden onset breathlessness and chest pains. On examination he is in pain, sweaty, has a tachycardia and BP was 90/50. ☐

THEME: BREATHLESSNESS

A   Pleural effusion
B   Inhalation of foreign body
C   Chronic Obstructive Pulmonary Disease
D   Anaemia
E   Pneumothorax
F   Laryngeal oedema
G   Pulmonary fibrosis
H   Asthma
I   Left ventricular failure
J   Bronchiectasis
K   Psychogenic breathlessness

For each scenario described below, select the most likely diagnosis from the list above. Each option may be used once, more than once or not at all.

6. A 77-year-old retired engineer complains of increasing breathlessness over several months. Examination shows diffuse fine inspiratory crepitations and clubbing.

7. A 29-year-old woman being treated with clomiphene for infertility complains of increasing breathlessness and abdominal distension over the last three weeks. She denies chest pain and has no previous respiratory history.

8. An 82-year-old lady with myelodysplasia has become progressively breathless over the last two weeks. Examination reveals a tachycardia.

9. One summer's afternoon you are called to the beach where a trainee scuba diver has collapsed. She apparently complained of sudden left-sided pain on surfacing. When you arrive she is unconscious and tachypnoeic. Examination reveals reduced breath sounds on the left.

10. A three-year-old boy suddenly becomes breathless while eating at a children's party. When you examine him he is coughing and spluttering with inspiratory wheeze.

11. A 92-year-old lady is found extremely breathless in the middle of the night. She prefers to sit upright and on examination she has an irregular pulse, basal crepitations and is cyanosed.

MULTIPLE BEST ANSWER QUESTIONS

1. **Which TWO statements about childhood asthma are true?**
   - ☐ **A**   Persistent cough may be the only symptom
   - ☐ **B**   About 50% of children will grow out of the disease
   - ☐ **C**   Outdoor exercises should be discouraged in winter months
   - ☐ **D**   Inhaled sodium cromoglycate is the drug of choice for prevention
   - ☐ **E**   Inhaled steroids normally stunt growth

2. **When discussing smoking which TWO statements are true?**
   - ☐ **A**   Non-smokers have a far greater risk of ischaemic heart disease if they live with a smoker
   - ☐ **B**   Nicotine replacement therapy is of no additional help in smoking cessation when the GP has given advice
   - ☐ **C**   The doctor-patient relationship may be harmed if the GP advises all smokers to stop smoking as part of a routine
   - ☐ **D**   The increase in smoking is mostly because of the increasing elderly population

3. **A severe asthma attack in an adult is characterised by which THREE indicators?**
   - ☐ **A**   Restricted daily activities
   - ☐ **B**   Peak flow rate of 70% of predicted value
   - ☐ **C**   Pulse rate of 110/min
   - ☐ **D**   Difficulty in speaking
   - ☐ **E**   Peripheral cyanosis

4. **Which TWO of the following are risk factors for the development of chronic obstructive pulmonary disease?**
   - ☐ **A**   Male sex
   - ☐ **B**   Working with aniline dyes
   - ☐ **C**   Low socio-economic status

5. **Which THREE statements apply to lung cancer?**
   - ☐ **A**   Causes deaths in the ratio 2:1 for men and women in the UK
   - ☐ **B**   Is most prevalent among people aged over 70 years
   - ☐ **C**   Is most commonly adenocarcinoma among smokers
   - ☐ **D**   Has a clear genetic association
   - ☐ **E**   Is associated with the level of urban pollution

6. **What THREE common conditions cause increased resonance?**
   - ☐ **A**   Empyema
   - ☐ **B**   Acute asthma
   - ☐ **C**   Pneumothorax
   - ☐ **D**   Emphysema
   - ☐ **E**   Lung cancer
   - ☐ **F**   Hyperventilation

SINGLE BEST ANSWER QUESTIONS

1. **Which ONE of the following is NOT a recognised association with finger clubbing?**
    - ☐ **A** Bronchiectasis
    - ☐ **B** Emphysema
    - ☐ **C** Lung cancer
    - ☐ **D** Hepatic cirrhosis
    - ☐ **E** Crohn's disease

2. **When using inhaled steroids in treatment, which ONE statement does NOT apply?**
    - ☐ **A** Side-effects are unusual at low doses
    - ☐ **B** Children with episodic wheezing associated with viral illness are included
    - ☐ **C** Systemic absorption takes place
    - ☐ **D** Fluticasone may have less systemic side-effects than beclomethasone
    - ☐ **E** High dosage can slow growth in children

3. **When considering treatment in chest infections, which ONE statement is true?**
    - ☐ **A** 25% of chest infections seen in General Practice are due to pneumonia
    - ☐ **B** 50% of patients with lower respiratory tract infections receive antibiotics in General Practice
    - ☐ **C** Antibiotics should not be delayed in patients with COPD

4. **Which ONE of the following statements about the investigations of asthma in children is true?**
    - ☐ **A** Skin allergy tests are often diagnostic of the precipitating cause
    - ☐ **B** Chest radiographs are indicated whenever there is an acute episode
    - ☐ **C** Pulmonary function tests are useful in children over 2 years of age
    - ☐ **D** FEV_1 is more reliable in demonstrating airways obstruction than peak expiratory flow

5. **Which of these is NOT a recognised cause of cough?**
    - ☐ **A** Inhaled foreign body
    - ☐ **B** Lisinopril
    - ☐ **C** Metformin
    - ☐ **D** Lung cancer
    - ☐ **E** Cardiac failure

6. **Which ONE of these statements apply in diagnosis of asthma?**
- [ ] **A** 15% reversibility by bronchial dilators is an essential diagnostic test
- [ ] **B** Cough is an important diagnostic feature
- [ ] **C** Once diagnosed as asthmatics, children remain asthmatic for the rest of their lives
- [ ] **D** Steroid inhalers have an immediate bronchial dilator effect
- [ ] **E** Family history of asthma is irrelevant

7. **Which ONE of the following statements does NOT apply to bronchial carcinoma?**
- [ ] **A** Screening is of little benefit
- [ ] **B** It is more common in urban areas
- [ ] **C** Nickel is a recognised risk factor
- [ ] **D** The incidence in females is rising
- [ ] **E** Haemoptysis suggests a poor prognosis

8. **In asthma which ONE of the following statements is true?**
- [ ] **A** Mortality has been falling steadily over the past ten years
- [ ] **B** The long-acting inhaled bronchodilators are recommended for first-line therapy
- [ ] **C** Bacterial infections are a common cause of acute attacks
- [ ] **D** More than 90% of patients have hyperreactive airways
- [ ] **E** Salbutamol and terbutaline act on adrenergic nerve endings to relax airway smooth muscle

ADMINISTRATION
AND MANAGEMENT
QUESTIONS

EXTENDED MATCHING QUESTIONS

THEME: LEGISLATION

A Access to Health Records Act 1990
B Access to Medical Reports Act 1988
C Data Protection Act 1984
D Disability Discrimination Act 1995
E Rehabilitation of Offenders Act 1974

For each of the descriptions, select the single most likely Act. Each option may be used once, more than once, or not at all.

1. After a certain length of time, criminal convictions must not be mentioned in any reports ☐

2. Patients can see any reports prepared for insurance companies ☐

3. Allows patients to see their own medical notes ☐

4. Gives employers responsibilities to employees who have previously been disabled ☐

5. Ensures that personal data is only held for specific purposes ☐

THEME: VOLUNTARY ORGANISATIONS

A Alanon
B ASH
C Compassionate Friends
D CRUSE
E Gingerbread
F Marie Curie Memorial Foundation
G MIND
H NSPCC
I RELATE
J RNIB
K RSPB
L RSPCA
M Terrence Higgins Trust
N Turning point

For each of the situations, select the single most appropriate organisation. Each option may be used once, more than once, or not at all.

6. Blindness ☐

7. Widows with bereavement problems ☐

8. Marriage problems ☐

9. Mental illness ☐

10. AIDS ☐

11. Bereaved parents ☐

12. Relatives of people with alcohol problems ☐

13. Child abuse ☐

14. One parent families ☐

15. Cancer ☐

16. Children suffering bereavement problems after death of parents ☐

17. Smokers ☐

18. Drug abuse ☐

THEME: MEDICAL CERTIFICATES

A Med 3
B Med 4
C Med 5
D Med 6
E Med 10
F DS 1500

For each of the descriptions, select the single most likely medical certificate. Each option may be used once, more than once, or not at all.

19. Issued when a vague diagnosis has been given on a certificate □

20. Is the usual certificate issued by a medical practitioner if a patient is off work because of sickness for more than seven days □

21. Is issued by a hospital if a patient is to be off work due to illness □

22. Is issued about a patient who has a terminal illness □

23. Is issued at the patient's request when personal capability assessment is being considered □

24. Can be issued for up to six months when the patient is first off work with an illness □

25. Can be issued as a sickness certificate on the basis of a written report from another doctor □

THEME: REGULATORY BODIES

A General Medical Council
B Joint Committee for Post Graduate Training in General Practice
C National Institute for Clinical Excellence
D Commission for Health Improvement
E National Clinical Assessment Authority
F United Kingdom Central Council (UKCC)
G Primary Care Trust
H Local Medical Committee

For each description below, select the most appropriate option from the list above. Each option may be used once, more than once or not at all

26. Aims to appraise new technologies, produce national guidelines and encourage quality improvement ☐

27. Will address concerns over underperformance and incompetence ☐

28. Will be responsible for holding and maintaining a list of approved non-principals from April 2002 ☐

29. Maintain a list of nurses and midwives who are eligible to practice ☐

30. Are responsible for maintaining a list of all vocationally trained general practitioners ☐

THEME: NUMBERS OF PEOPLE ON A GP'S LIST

A 5
B 10
C 25
D 50
E 100
F 200

For each of the groups of people below, select the single most likely numbers. Each option may be used once, more than once, or not at all.

31. Number of unemployed people ☐

32. Number of schizophrenic patients ☐

33. Number of deaf people ☐

34. Number of people receiving state benefit ☐

35. Number of blind people ☐

THEME: GP INCOME

A Capitation fees
B Basic Practice Allowance
C Immediately necessary treatment fee
D Minor Surgery fee
E Registration fees
F Health Promotion Clinics
G Target immunisations for children
H Postgraduate education allowance
I Immunisation item of service fees
J Night visit fee
K Temporary resident fee
L Emergency treatment fee

From the list of options below, select the most appropriate option from the list above.

36. Payable for a medical examination within three months of joining the practice ☐

37. Payable for certain travel vaccinations ☐

38. May be claimed for telephone advice after 10 pm ☐

39. Paid for providing a service in an emergency to a person whose stay in the area will be less than 24 hours ☐

40. Payable for patients resident in the area more than three months, refused acceptance on list and not on list of a local GP ☐

MULTIPLE BEST ANSWER QUESTIONS

1. **Select THREE restrictions with respect to driving which apply to patients at risk of having seizures**
   - ☐ **A**   Patients are obliged to contact the DVLA if they believe themselves to be at risk of seizures
   - ☐ **B**   A patient's doctor is obliged to inform the DVLA of a patient at risk of seizures
   - ☐ **C**   A patient may continue to drive following a single nocturnal seizure
   - ☐ **D**   A recent diagnosis of cerebral glioma prohibits driving
   - ☐ **E**   A recent diagnosis of bronchogenic carcinoma prohibits driving

2. **Select TWO occupations suitable for someone with a history of epilepsy, but not fit for the last five years**
   - ☐ **A**   An aircraft pilot
   - ☐ **B**   A prison officer
   - ☐ **C**   A teacher
   - ☐ **D**   A train driver
   - ☐ **E**   An army officer
   - ☐ **F**   A merchant seafarer

3. **Select THREE of the following. Burnout in General Practitioners is**
   - ☐ **A**   more likely to be found in doctors with postgraduate qualifications
   - ☐ **B**   less likely in those who attend postgraduate meetings
   - ☐ **C**   unrelated to depression
   - ☐ **D**   more likely in doctors with obsessional personalities
   - ☐ **E**   more likely in those with high personal standards
   - ☐ **F**   less likely in those who are reluctant to delegate at work

4. **Select THREE factors concerning heartsink patients**
   - ☐ **A**   Doctors with postgraduate medical qualifications have more heartsink patients
   - ☐ **B**   Doctors trained in counselling have more heartsink patients
   - ☐ **C**   The more heartsink patients seen the lower the job satisfaction
   - ☐ **D**   Heartsink patients have high rates of non-attendance for appointments
   - ☐ **E**   About 1/3 of heartsink patients have a serious medical diagnosis

5. **Which THREE of the following are available as over-the-counter medicine and do not need a doctor's prescription?**
   - ☐ **A**   Cimetidine
   - ☐ **B**   Piroxicam tablets
   - ☐ **C**   Ibuprofen tablets
   - ☐ **D**   Topical acyclovir
   - ☐ **E**   Co-proxamol

6. **Free NHS prescriptions are available to which THREE groups of patients?**
☐ **A** All patients with thyrotoxicosis
☐ **B** All patients with myasthenia gravis
☐ **C** All patients with diabetes
☐ **D** Patients with permanent fistula
☐ **E** Patients with epilepsy

7. **Select THREE statements about Advance directives**
☐ **A** Once made, cannot be withdrawn
☐ **B** Need to state that death might result from the directive
☐ **C** Must not be deliberately ignored
☐ **D** Need to be signed and witnessed
☐ **E** Can stop the administration of oral nutrition and hydration

8. **Under the Terms of Service for GPs, which THREE of these apply to a full-time principal?**
☐ **A** Need only be available for 26 hours a week
☐ **B** Hours of availability have to be over the five days in a week
☐ **C** Must be available (in person or by use of a deputy) 24 hours a day
☐ **D** Can only take a maximum of ten weeks' holiday per year
☐ **E** Must claim for contraception (e.g. GMS4 cervical smear targets and capitation payments

9. **Select THREE Items of Service payments**
☐ **A** Cervical smears
☐ **B** All immunisations
☐ **C** Contraception
☐ **D** Night visits
☐ **E** Maternity work

10. **On confirmation of death, one needs to inform the coroner about which THREE of these studies?**
☐ **A** Patient was not seen in the previous 14 days
☐ **B** Death followed a termination of pregnancy
☐ **C** Patient has had chemotherapy in the last month
☐ **D** Patient has a pacemaker fitted
☐ **E** Death was due to an industrial disease

11. **Which THREE statements apply to GPs working under the Personal Medical Services (PMS) system as opposed to General Medical Services (GMS)?**
☐ **A** Are bound by regulations in the red book
☐ **B** Have a cash-limited contract
☐ **C** Can employ salaried GPs
☐ **D** Can be paid for more secondary care work done in primary care
☐ **E** Have increased job security

12. **Select TWO of the following statements which apply to a principal in General Practice under General Medical Services**
- [ ] **A** Is not responsible for the acts of the assistants in the practice
- [ ] **B** Who is in partnership, must receive not less than a quarter of a share of the partner with the greatest share
- [ ] **C** Will automatically get a postgraduate education allowance
- [ ] **D** Will automatically get a seniority allowance, after seven years in practice
- [ ] **E** Cannot stop being responsible for their patients, 24 hours a day, seven days a week

13. **With regard to General Practice premises, select TWO of the following:**
- [ ] **A** The majority of General Practitioners are based in Health Centres
- [ ] **B** They are not required to meet the standards set in the Disability Discrimination Act
- [ ] **C** If owner-occupied, can receive help in the form of an improvement grant
- [ ] **D** Can be used for private work as long as it does not bring in more than 20% of the total income
- [ ] **E** Are reviewed by the District Valuer's Office every three years, for rental purposes

14. **The red book (statement of fees and allowances) states TWO of the following:**
- [ ] **A** Quality payment may be automatically paid to training practices
- [ ] **B** A prescribing incentive scheme should be made available
- [ ] **C** Doctors can work as retainees for up to four sessions in a single practice
- [ ] **D** An assistance allowance is available, irrespective of the list size
- [ ] **E** Minor surgery payment is dependent on the number of principals in the practice and the list size

15. **Select the THREE items which can be prescribed on FP10**
- [ ] **A** Viagra tablets
- [ ] **B** Pen insulin injection devices
- [ ] **C** Neck collar
- [ ] **D** Blood pricking lancets
- [ ] **E** Panadol

16. **A patient requests access to their records. Which TWO of the following are true?**
- [ ] **A** Paper notes about an individual are the legal property of that individual
- [ ] **B** Under the Medical Records Act 1988 a doctor must amend a report before sending it if the patient disagrees with it
- [ ] **C** If a patient requests a copy of a medical report, the practice may make a charge for this
- [ ] **D** Medical records must be divulged in full should a patient request this
- [ ] **E** Patients may view a copy of the report up to six months after it has been written.
- [ ] **F** Medical records are exempt from the Data Protection Act
- [ ] **G** GPs may only charge for access to paper records, not computer records

SINGLE BEST ANSWER QUESTIONS

1. **Most commercial flights will allow pregnant women to fly on board up to which ONE of gestational periods given below?**
   - ☐ **A** 38 weeks
   - ☐ **B** 34 weeks
   - ☐ **C** 30 weeks
   - ☐ **D** 26 weeks

2. **Core General Practitioner's Service Contract covers which ONE of the following?**
   - ☐ **A** Provision of family planning services
   - ☐ **B** Issuing national insurance certificate form Med 3
   - ☐ **C** Carrying out an annual health check
   - ☐ **D** Seeing all patients over the age of 75 on an annual basis
   - ☐ **E** Provision of minor surgery services

3. **Which ONE of the following is NOT correct regarding computerised Medical Records?**
   - ☐ **A** It is legal for GPs not to have to write medical records in cards provided by the Secretary of State
   - ☐ **B** Allows items-of-service claims to be done electronically
   - ☐ **C** Have been proven to lead to poorer consultations
   - ☐ **D** Studies have shown that nurses are better at data entry than doctors
   - ☐ **E** Are not admissible as evidence in a court of law

4. **Which ONE of these does NOT apply to Personal Medical Services (PMS)?**
   - ☐ **A** Allows greater flexibility in provision of general medical services
   - ☐ **B** Has to have a cash limited prescribing budget associated
   - ☐ **C** Allows employment of salaried doctors
   - ☐ **D** Can allow nurses, or community trusts, to employ doctors to provide personal medical services
   - ☐ **E** PMS plus allows provision of secondary care services in primary care

5. **A 32-year-old lady with an established diagnosis of bipolar affective disorder is visited regularly by an outreach team. The team is increasingly concerned about her self-care since she stopped taking her mood stabilising drugs. If she needs to be detained in hospital, which SINGLE section of the Mental Health Act (1983) would be the MOST appropriate?**
   - ☐ **A** Section 2
   - ☐ **B** Section 3
   - ☐ **C** Section 4
   - ☐ **D** Section 5
   - ☐ **E** Section 7

6. **Which ONE of the following would the General Medical Council not expect a Doctor to do?**
    - ☐ A   Be actively supportive of the professional development of each member of their practice team
    - ☐ B   Report another doctor immediately if patients are at risk of harm
    - ☐ C   Meet performance targets set by management
    - ☐ D   Disclose personal information about a patient if this is in the wider public interest, after weighing up the harm and benefit
    - ☐ E   Be prepared to explain and justify their decisions

7. **Which ONE of the following is true concerning NHS Direct?**
    - ☐ A   Is part of a GP out-of-hours co-operative service
    - ☐ B   Is usually run by nurses
    - ☐ C   Has been shown to be cost effective
    - ☐ D   Has Crown immunity
    - ☐ E   Is preferred by patients, over advice given by their GPs

8. **You are a new principal, having just completed VTS training. The practice manager asks you for your CME certificates to claim your PGEA allowance. Which ONE of the following is true regarding PGEA?**
    - ☐ A   Only attendance at approved courses is eligible for PGEA
    - ☐ B   Vocational training allows the principal to claim the full allowance for the first three years after completing their training
    - ☐ C   No more than 10 days' CME may be claimed per year
    - ☐ D   Personal Learning Plans may be accepted for PGEA if approved by the clinical tutor
    - ☐ E   All costs involved in undertaking CME may be reclaimed from the PCT

9. **Your practice needs new premises. Select the SINGLE best answer from the following statements regarding financing.**
    - ☐ A   Financing under the cost rent scheme involves the partnership paying the interest while the FHSA pays off the capital sum
    - ☐ B   The cost rent scheme allows the practice to use the surgery for private practice as long as the rental income does not exceed 25% of the monthly FHSA payment
    - ☐ C   When financing under the cost-rent scheme, the interest rate on the loan is fixed for the life of the agreement and cannot be changed
    - ☐ D   Private Finance Initiative funding involves a private company building and maintaining the surgery, for which the practice then pays a rental fee.
    - ☐ E   For practices operating under a PMS contract, money is available for re-development of existing premises.

10. Regarding drugs carried in a GP's bag, which ONE of the following statements is true?

☐ **A**   When administering drugs to a patient in an emergency, a prescription can be made out in their name which is then used to replenish your stocks

☐ **B**   No dispensing fee is payable for patients who live within 1.5 miles of a pharmacy

☐ **C**   Drugs must be purchased by the GP, and reimbursement claimed from the FHSA at the end of the month.

☐ **D**   GPs may choose not to carry controlled drugs if they feel this places them at risk of mugging or burglary

☐ **E**   If controlled drugs are kept in the front of a car, the car must be locked at all times

11. With regard to complaints made to a practice, which ONE of the following statements is true?

☐ **A**   The time limit for a patient to lodge a complaint is six months

☐ **B**   Complaints must be acknowledged within seven working days

☐ **C**   The senior partner is responsible for the administration of the complaints system

☐ **D**   90% of practice complaints are because of rudeness or other interpersonal issues

☐ **E**   There must be a written response within 10 working days

RESEARCH, EPIDEMIOLOGY AND STATISTICS QUESTIONS

EXTENDED MATCHING QUESTIONS

THEME: XENICAL

A 1
B 2
C 2.5
D 3
E 5
F 6
G 10
H 15
I 25
J 28
K 30
L 32
M 35
N Breathlessness
O Aerobics
P Dietary
Q Will power
R Activity
S Hypothyroidism
T Hypertension
U Gastroesophageal reflux

From the list of options, select the appropriate word for each missing gap. Each option may be used once, more than once or not at all.

"The National Institute for Clinical Excellence has recommended that orlistat should be prescribed under the following conditions:

– only for individuals with a body mass index (BMI) of (**1**) kg/m^2 or more (and no associated co-morbidity) or for individuals with a BMI of (**2**) or more in the presence of other risk factors (e.g. type 2 diabetes (**3**) hypercholesterolaemia)

– only for individuals who have lost at least (**4**) kg body weight by (**5**) control and increased (**6**) in the preceding month

– only for individuals aged between 18 and 75 years

– treatment should continue beyond three months only if weight loss is greater than (**7**) % from start of treatment

– treatment should continue beyond (**8**) months only if weight loss is greater than (**9**) % from start of treatment

– treatment should not usually continue beyond (**10**) year(s) and never beyond (**11**) year(s)".

THEME: STATISTICS

A   112/183
B   112/175
C   112/1000
D   71/183
E   71/825
F   71/1000
G   63/175
H   63/817
I   63/1000
J   754/817
K   754/825
L   754/1000

1000 patients were tested in General Practice for colonic cancer using a new test. The test was positive in 112 patients who actually had the disease, and 71 patients who did not have the disease. The test was negative in 63 patients who actually did have the disease and in 754 patients who did not have the disease.

For each of the statements, select the single most likely option. Each option can be used once, more than once, or not at all.

12. What is the sensitivity? ☐

13. What is the positive predictive value? ☐

14. What is the negative predictive value? ☐

15. What is the specificity? ☐

THEME: TRIALS

A   Case control study
B   Cohort study
C   Correlation study
D   Descriptive study
E   Meta-analysis study
F   Randomised clinical trial
G   Randomised cross-over trial
H   Randomised double blind placebo-controlled trial

For each description below, select the single most likely study. Each option may be used once, more than once, or not at all.

16. A survey to find the prevalence of diabetes in a General Practice population ☐

17. A study looking at the previous use of aspirin in patients with DVTs and healthy patients ☐

18. The prevention of DVTs was studied in air travellers who were assigned randomly to receive either stockings or exercise ☐

19. Reported national incidence of psychotic illness is found to be associated with the national seizure of illicit drugs ☐

20. The results of several investigations into exposure to vibrating machinery and the development of HAVS are combined to reach a conclusion ☐

THEME: STATISTICAL TERMS

A 0
B 1
C Just over 1
D Just under 2
E 2
F Just over 2
G Just under 3
H 3
I Over 3

The number of receptionists employed by General Practices in a local area was as follows:

1,2,0,7,0,4,2,2,1,1,2.

For each of the questions, select the single most likely option. Each option can be used once, more than once, or not at all.

21. What is the mean? ☐

22. What is the median? ☐

23. What is the mode? ☐

THEME: ECONOMICS

A Cost
B Cost benefit analysis
C Cost benefit ratio
D Cost effective
E Cost effectiveness analysis
F Cost effectiveness ratio
G Cost minimisation analysis
H Cost of illness analysis
I Cost utility analysis
J Price

For each of the statements, select the single most likely option. Each of the options can be used once, more than once, or not at all.

24. A type of economic assessment in which both cost and benefit are expressed in monetary terms ☐

25. The monetary value of the resources consumed in its production or delivery ☐

26. The ratio of total cost of an intervention divided by the gain in selected health outcome (e.g. cost per life/year gained) ☐

27. A study to estimate the economic burden of a particular disease ☐

28. A study to assess the benefit of an intervention e.g. quality-adjusted life-year ☐

THEME: STUDIES

A Case control study
B Cohort study
C Correlation study
D Descriptive
E Meta-analysis
F Randomised double blind cross-over trial
G Randomised double blind placebo-controlled trial

For each of these descriptions, select the single most likely study. Each option can be used once, more than once, or not at all.

29. A group of children using mobile phones was matched with a group only using land-based phones. The groups were both followed up looking at the incidence of brain tumours.

30. Patients with osteoarthritis were randomly given drug A or drug B which looked identical. The clinical condition was monitored. The patients were then given the alternative drug and monitored again. Neither the doctor nor the patient knew which drug was being taken at each time.

31. Patients with warts were randomly given preparation X in a paste base, or the paste base alone. The warty lesions were observed. Neither the doctor nor the patient knew which treatment was being given.

32. A group of patients with DVTs was matched with a healthy group of people of the same age, sex and social class. It was then established how often they had travelled by plane in the last year.

33. A group of diabetics was investigated to see if the mothers had had certain infections during the pregnancies

THEME: SCREENING TESTS

A 0.2
B 0.8
C 20%
D 25%
E 33%
F 50%
G 66%
H 80%
I 93%

In a sample of 100 undergoing a screening test, there were 20 true positives, 5 false negatives, 5 false positives and 70 true negatives.

For each option, select the single most likely percentage. Each option may be used once, more than once, or not at all.

34. Sensitivity ☐

35. Specificity ☐

36. Prevalence ☐

37. Predictive value ☐

38. Yield ☐

THEME: RESEARCH METHODS

A Clinical audit
B Longitudinal study
C Observational study
D Qualitative study
E Randomised controlled trial
F Survey

For each of the statements, select the single most likely option. Each option can be used once, more than once, or not at all.

39. A General Practice wishes to see how it manages its diabetic patients as compared to other practices in the area ☐

40. A Health Authority wishes to know how many of its black African population is screened for sickle-cell ☐

41. A General Practice wishes to explore the views of women who do not wish to breast feed ☐

42. A GP wishes to find out if Salbutamol inhaler is less effective than brand-named Ventolin ☐

43. An occupational health doctor wishes to find out if telling the factory workers they have hypertension leads to more time off sick ☐

THEME: STATISTICAL TERMS

A Sensitivity
B Sensitivity analysis
C Significance levels
D Specificity
E Standard deviation
F Standard error of the mean (SEM)
G Standard normal variant
H Standardised mortality rate

For each of the statements, select the single most likely option. Each option can be used once, more than once, or not at all

44. A term used for describing recomputation of results using different parameters, values or perspectives to investigate whether any conclusions drawn are altered as a result ☐

45. A measure of the spread of a distribution and is equal to the square root of the variance ☐

46. The true positive ratio, that is, the proportion of patients with disease who return a positive test ☐

47. Widely used statistic to describe the precision associated with the estimate of the mean ☐

48. Mortality rate adjusted to take account of the composition of the population to which it refers ☐

THEME: THE FOLLOWING LITERATURE RELATES TO MODELS OF THE CONSULTATION IN GENERAL PRACTICE

A Stott CP, Davis RH. *The exceptional potential in each primary care consultation*. JRCGP 1979; 29: 201–5.
B Pendleton D, *The consultation*, Oxford, 1984.
C Berne E, *Transactional analysis – Games people play*, Penguin, 1970.
D Heron J, *Human potential research project*, Univ of Surrey, 1975.
E Balint M, *The doctor, his patient and the illness*, London Tavistock, 1958.
F Byrne PS, Long BEL, *Doctors talking to patients*, DHSS, 1976.
G Neighbour R, *The Inner Consultation*, Petroc Press, 1999.

Each of the following comments relate to consultation texts above, select the single most likely reference. Each option can be used once, more than once or not at all.

49. The Seven Tasks ☐

50. Modification of help-seeking behaviour ☐

51. Six logical phases to a consultation ☐

52. Doctor as drug ☐

53. To achieve a shared understanding of the problems with the patient ☐

54. Parent, adult and child ego states ☐

55. Cathartic ☐

56. Opportunistic health promotion ☐

57. Safety-netting ☐

58. Apostolic function ☐

THEME: A YEAR IN GENERAL PRACTICE

A 500
B 200
C 25
D 10
E <1

For each of the conditions, select the most likely number of patients consulting with each condition. Each option may be used once, more than once, or not at all.

59. Chronic renal failure ☐

60. Chronic mental illness ☐

61. Hypertension ☐

62. Thyroid disease ☐

63. Diabetes ☐

THEME: TRIALS CONCERNING CORONARY HEART DISEASE

A   4S
B   ASSET
C   CARE Study
D   GISSI
E   GREAT Group Study
F   ISIS-2
G   Nurses Study

For each description below, select the most likely trial. Each option may be used once, more than once, or not at all.

64. A trial of thrombolytic therapy using streptokinase controlled against placebo   ☐

65. A trial of pre-hospital thrombolytic treatment   ☐

66. This trial used simvastatin   ☐

67. This was a large-scale trial of lipid-lowering drugs in secondary prevention; pravastatin was the active drug used   ☐

68. A trial of thrombolytic therapy using aspirin and/or streptokinase   ☐

69. Study involved the use of unopposed oestrogens   ☐

70. Trial of a thrombolytic therapy used alteplase   ☐

THEME: CARDIOVASCULAR TRIALS

A SOLVD-T
B UKPDS-1998
C 4S
D HOPE
E ISIS-2
F WOSCOPS
G CARE
H Antiplatelet Trialists Collaboration 94
I HOT

For each of the following descriptions of clinical trials, choose the corresponding trial from the list above. Each option may be used once, more than once or not at all.

71. Confirmed the value of primary prevention in preventing cardiovascular deaths in patients with hyperlipidaemia ☐

72. Confirmed the value of treating patients post MI with left ventricular dysfunction with ACE inhibitors ☐

73. Showed the benefit of secondary prevention in patients with ischaemic heart disease with normal lipid levels ☐

74. Confirmed the value of immediate aspirin after MI ☐

75. Confirmed that the ideal BP in terms of reducing cardiovascular complications is 140/80 ☐

76. Confirmed the value of tight control of blood pressure in diabetes ☐

THEME: HYPERTENSION

A 110
B 100
C 145
D 150
E 160
F Non-pharmacological measures
G 5
H 15
I 10
J 85
K 90
L Pharmacological measures
M 100
N ACE inhibitors
O Thiazides
P Aspirin
Q Beta blockers
R Fibrates
S Clopidogrel
T Statins

Below is a summary of the British Hypertension Society Guidelines (2000). For each omitted item, select the most appropriate option from the list above.

*Use **(77)** in all hypertensive and borderline hypertensive people*

*Initiate antihypertensive drug treatment in people with sustained systolic blood pressure 160 mmHg or sustained diastolic blood pressure **(78)** mmHg*

*Decide on treatment in people with sustained systolic blood pressure between 140 and 159 mmHg or sustained diastolic blood pressure between 90 and 99 mmHg according to the presence or absence of target organ damage, cardiovascular disease, diabetes, or a 10 year coronary heart disease risk **(79)** % according to the Joint British Societies coronary heart disease risk assessment programme or risk chart*

*Optimal blood pressure treatment targets are systolic blood pressure < **(80)** mmHg and diastolic blood pressure < **(81)** mmHg; the minimum acceptable level of control (audit standard) recommended is < **(82)** / < **(83)** mmHg*

*In the absence of contraindications or compelling indications for other antihypertensive agents, **(84)** or **(85)** are preferred as first line treatment for the majority of hypertensive people; compelling indications and contraindications for all antihypertensive drug classes are specified*

*Other drugs that reduce cardiovascular risk must also be considered; these include **(86)** and **(87)***

MULTIPLE BEST ANSWER QUESTIONS

1. **Select THREE of these statements concerning mental health of children and adolescents in Great Britain**
    - ☐ **A**   10% of 5 to 15-year-olds have a clinically significant mental disorder
    - ☐ **B**   More girls are affected
    - ☐ **C**   More children are affected in families with both parents working
    - ☐ **D**   30% of children with a mental disorder have no contact with General Practice or specialist services
    - ☐ **E**   These children are three times more likely to have special educational needs

2. **Select TWO statements that relate most to children in social class V compared with social class I**
    - ☐ **A**   Are four times more likely to die in an accident
    - ☐ **B**   Are taller in height
    - ☐ **C**   Have the same rate of chronic illness
    - ☐ **D**   Have a much higher infant mortality rate

3. **Select TWO of the following statements regarding obesity in the UK**
    - ☐ **A**   Is increasing in prevalence
    - ☐ **B**   Is more common in social class I compared to social class V
    - ☐ **C**   Should be treated with pharmacological intervention when the BMI is 29
    - ☐ **D**   The body fat distribution in the South Asian population is the same as that in the white population
    - ☐ **E**   Is an independent risk factor for hypertension

4. **The risk of dying from liver cirrhosis is higher than average in which TWO groups?**
    - ☐ **A**   Farm workers
    - ☐ **B**   Journalists
    - ☐ **C**   Medical practitioners
    - ☐ **D**   Printing machine minders
    - ☐ **E**   Managers in the building and contracting trade

5. **Select THREE correct items concerning the National Service Framework (NSF) on Cardiovascular disease**
    - ☐ **A**   Is limited to the National Health Service
    - ☐ **B**   Specialist smoking cessation clinics are recommended in General Practice setting
    - ☐ **C**   Has specific targets on the number of revascularisation operations
    - ☐ **D**   Expects General Practice to have a disease register of all their patients who have had an ischaemic heart disease
    - ☐ **E**   Requires cardiac rehabilitation to be offered to all patients

6. **When comparing retrospective studies to prospective studies, select THREE statements relating to retrospective studies**
□ **A** More prone to bias
□ **B** More expensive
□ **C** Less attributable to cause and effect
□ **D** Quicker to do
□ **E** More rigorous

7. **In the trial of two anti-epileptic drugs following head injury 18 out of 27 patients treated by drug A were fit free one month after injury compared with 5 out of 17 patients treated with drug B. Select THREE of the following statements which apply if the significance of these results is tested by the chi-squared test**
□ **A** The figures should first be converted to percentages
□ **B** The test is non-parametric
□ **C** There is one degree of freedom
□ **D** A value of chi-squared of 4.3 would imply that the result would have been obtained by chance in 43 out of 100 trials
□ **E** The results would be invalidated if most of the cases treated with drug A had developed epilepsy immediately after the head injury compared with those treated with drug B

8. **Select THREE of the following statements. Systematic reviews**
□ **A** are dependent on having good randomised controlled trials
□ **B** odds ratios and associated 95% confidence intervals are usually reported
□ **C** are available for most medical interventions
□ **D** are routinely used by commissioners to make purchasing decisions
□ **E** can sometimes lead to wrong conclusions

9. **Which TWO of the following are true?**
□ **A** The annual prevalence of a condition reflects the number of new cases reported annually
□ **B** Cohort studies are generally used to study a group of subjects with a particular disease and compare them with normal controls
□ **C** In a frequency distribution, the mode is the most frequently observed value
□ **D** If a measurement has a skewed distribution, then the mean and mode are always different
□ **E** The standard deviation of population may be smaller than the standard error of a sample mean from that population

10. **Choose THREE of these statements. The standard deviation of a group of observations**

☐ **A**   is the square of the variance of the group
☐ **B**   is a measure of the scatter of the observations around the mean
☐ **C**   is a valid statistical parameter only if the observations have a normal distribution
☐ **D**   is numerically higher than the standard error of the mean
☐ **E**   may be used as a basis for the calculation of chi-squared

11. **Which THREE of the following are correct statements about statistical items?**

☐ **A** $P = 0.01$ is a lower degree of statistical significance than $p = 0.05$
☐ **B**   The prevalence of ischaemic heart disease varies in different areas of the UK
☐ **C**   In a frequency distribution the mode is the most frequently observed value
☐ **D**   The median is the point on a scale of values which exactly divides the number of values into upper and lower halves
☐ **E**   The incidence of a disorder means the number suffering from that disorder at any one time

12. **The diastolic blood pressure readings of 1000 9-year-old children were found to have a statistically normal distribution with a mean value of 61 mmHg and a standard deviation of 8 mmHg. Which THREE of the following statements can be made about this study?**

☐ **A**   The mean and standard deviation completely define the distribution of diastolic blood pressure for this age group
☐ **B**   The mean diastolic blood pressure for this sample is equal to that of the whole population
☐ **C**   95% of the sample data lie within an interval defined by the mean +/- 2 standard deviations (i.e. The range 45–77 mmHg)
☐ **D**   The median is 53 (i.e. 1 standard deviation below the mean)
☐ **E**   The variance is 64 (i.e. The square of the standard deviation)

13. **A new antibiotic Z is compared with amoxycillin in a clinical trial. A higher proportion of those patients treated with Z respond in a given time (chi-squared 4.2; p <0.05). Which TWO of the following statements are true?**

☐ **A**   The improved response to Z is clinically significant
☐ **B**   Treatment with Z cannot be worse than treatment with amoxycillin
☐ **C**   The results would be invalidated if there was a significant difference in the ages of the two treatment groups
☐ **D**   The trial implies that a difference in response of 4.2 times was observed
☐ **E**   The results may have occurred by chance one time in twenty

14. **In the clinical trial of a new treatment, which THREE statements apply?**
- [ ] **A** The null hypothesis is true if there are significant differences between the response of the treatment and placebo group
- [ ] **B** The patients should be randomised
- [ ] **C** Stratum matching of patients is necessary if the groups are small
- [ ] **D** In a type one error the null hypothesis is wrongly rejected
- [ ] **E** The number of subjects required decreases as the power of the trial increases

15. **For the correlation coefficient r, which TWO of the following statements are correct?**
- [ ] **A** The value of r lies between –1 and +1
- [ ] **B** If r = 0.1 this excludes a significant correlation between the variables
- [ ] **C** If r is negative, one value increases while the other decreases
- [ ] **D** r would be useful in comparing the relationship between blood pressure and cardiovascular mortality in a population
- [ ] **E** It can be used to predict one variable from the value of the other

16. **The time taken to walk 10 metres was recorded in 50 patients who had suffered a stroke. The observations were found to be distributed symmetrically about the mean (47 seconds). Which THREE statements apply?**
- [ ] **A** The observations, being symmetrical about the mean, must follow a normal distribution
- [ ] **B** If the observations had been found to be positively skewed, their mode would have been less than the mean
- [ ] **C** The median time to walk 10 metres is equal to the 50th percentile
- [ ] **D** Computing the variance of the observations would provide a measure of their spread about the mean.
- [ ] **E** Computing the standard deviation of the observations would provide a measure of the reliability of the mean

17. **When looking at the referral rate to hospital specialists, which TWO of these are true?**
- [ ] **A** The greatest variation source is the GP
- [ ] **B** Deprivation accounts for about one-third of the difference in referral rates
- [ ] **C** GP experience in a specialty decreases the rate of referral
- [ ] **D** Prescribing rate goes down as referral rate rises
- [ ] **E** The smallest referral rate is in the largest practices

18. **Select THREE of the following concerning a GP with 2000 patients over a one year period. A GP will see:**
- [ ] **A** 21 cases of myocardial infarction
- [ ] **B** 12 cases of pneumonia
- [ ] **C** 32 cases of severe depression
- [ ] **D** 8 cases of new cancers
- [ ] **E** 6 patients with acute stroke

19. Select TWO items about the Oxcheck study

- ☐ **A**   Looked at secondary prevention in coronary artery disease
- ☐ **B**   Involved intensive, doctor-led intervention clinics in General Practice
- ☐ **C**   Showed that clinics were expensive and the results of prevention strategy were disappointing
- ☐ **D**   Moved focus to secondary prevention

20. The UK Prospective Diabetes Study Group showed which THREE of the following statements?

- ☐ **A**   Metformin is effective in overweight patients
- ☐ **B**   The combination of metformin and a sulphonylurea was associated with a slight increase in mortality
- ☐ **C**   Good blood pressure control did not reduce diabetic-related deaths
- ☐ **D**   Metformin was associated with less weight gain than other treatments
- ☐ **E**   Intensive control of blood glucose levels did not reduce microvascular complications

SINGLE BEST ANSWER QUESTIONS

1. Which ONE of the following is most true of strokes?
- ☐ **A** Are the commonest cause of disability in the UK
- ☐ **B** Are the commonest cause of death in the UK
- ☐ **C** About 20% of strokes are due to cerebral infarction
- ☐ **D** Each stroke episode has a 5% mortality
- ☐ **E** 50% of strokes recur in the next year

2. Select ONE statement. Hypertension Society guidelines:
- ☐ **A** look at end point trials with prevention of events
- ☐ **B** suggest that most patients can be managed on one drug alone
- ☐ **C** suggest optimal treatment levels are <150/<90
- ☐ **D** suggest optimal levels are achievable with a good practice register
- ☐ **E** suggest that non-pharmacological advice is of little value in long-term follow-up

3. According to 1999 British Hypertension Society Guidelines
- ☐ **A** A patient with blood pressure of 138/88 should be reviewed yearly
- ☐ **B** Suggested optional blood pressure target should be <150/<90 mmHg
- ☐ **C** A patient over the age of 80 should not be treated to the same extent as a patient aged 65
- ☐ **D** With a blood pressure reading of 160/100 in a patient aged 65, treatment should be started after one further reading
- ☐ **E** A patient with blood pressure of 220/110 with no papilloedema should be started on treatment immediately

4. A study finds that the height of a child compared with its siblings has values of r = 0.6 p<0.001. Which ONE of the following is true?
- ☐ **A** r is the correlation coefficient of probability
- ☐ **B** If p<0.001 it means that the result is highly significant
- ☐ **C** If p<0.001 it means that too few measurements have been made
- ☐ **D** If r <1 then a negative correlation exists
- ☐ **E** There is a definite linear relationship

5. Which ONE of these statements is NOT true in a normal (Gaussian) distribution?
- ☐ **A** The mode is the most frequent observation
- ☐ **B** The median divides the distribution exactly into two halves
- ☐ **C** The mean, median and the mode are numerically the same
- ☐ **D** The distribution is numerically the same as a poisson distribution
- ☐ **E** All the people in the sample are normal

6. **The median is used in preference to the arithmetic mean when which ONE of these applies?**
- ☐ **A** The variance is large
- ☐ **B** The sample size is small
- ☐ **C** The observations are from a population with a skew distribution
- ☐ **D** Observer error is likely to be large
- ☐ **E** Chi-squared is to be calculated

7. **An article in a medical journal states that in a study of gestational age at birth and neurological development at 12 months of age, r was found to be +0.56 and p<0.001. Which statement is correct?**
- ☐ **A** r is the correlation coefficient of probability
- ☐ **B** There is a negative association between gestational age and neurological development
- ☐ **C** There is a significant relationship between gestational age and neurological development
- ☐ **D** Pre-term birth causes an inhibition in neurological development
- ☐ **E** The small value of p means that too few infants were studied

8. **In the UK, respiratory diseases account for**
- ☐ **A** ¼ of medical admissions
- ☐ **B** 1 in 10 deaths
- ☐ **C** 1 in 10 working days lost through illness

9. **What is the commonest diagnosis leading to wheelchair use in the UK?**
- ☐ **A** Arthritis
- ☐ **B** Cerebrovascular disease
- ☐ **C** COAD
- ☐ **D** IHD
- ☐ **E** Amputation
- ☐ **F** Cancer

10. **In intermittent claudication, which ONE of the following statements is not correct?**
- ☐ **A** The clinical course is more benign in women than in men
- ☐ **B** Symptoms usually steadily deteriorate following presentation
- ☐ **C** Life expectancy is shorter than in unaffected individuals
- ☐ **D** Regular exercise improves blood flow in the long-term

11. **Data from the Framingham study**
- ☐ **A** Can be used to assess the rate of cerebrovascular disease in British men and women
- ☐ **B** Are useful in secondary prevention
- ☐ **C** Gives a useful indication of risk in any population
- ☐ **D** Do not apply to people with familial hyperlipidaemia
- ☐ **E** Involved about 5000 people

ANSWERS

MEDICINE
ANSWERS

CARDIOVASCULAR

EXTENDED MATCHING QUESTIONS

THEME: PULSES

1. **E** Plateau
2. **F** Pulsus alternans
3. **C** Collapsing
4. **B** Bisferiens
5. **F** Pulsus alternans
6. **D** Pulsus paradoxus
7. **D** Pulsus paradoxus
8. **E** Plateau

Plateau pulse is found in aortic stenosis, it is of low amplitude and has a slow rise and fall. Collapsing or water hammer pulse is found in aortic regurgitation. Pulsus alternans is found in left ventricular failure; there are alternate large and small amplitude beats, and it is usually found when taking blood pressure. A doubling in rate is noted as the mercury level falls.

Bisferiens is a double topped pulse, found in mixed aortic stenosis and regurgitation. Pulsus paradoxus is found in cardiac tamponade, severe COPD and the volume decreases markedly with inspiration.

THEME: ECG FINDINGS

9. **H** Short PR interval
10. **A** Absent P waves with ragged baseline
11. **F** Peaked T wave
12. **C** Large R waves in V1–V2
13. **I** Short QT interval
14. **G** Prolonged PR interval
15. **B** Inverted T wave
16. **E** Long QT interval
17. **D** Large S waves in V1–V2

ECG changes can be important and you will need to be aware of them. Right ventricular hypertrophy can result in large R waves in V1–V2 and large S waves in V5–V6. Similarly, left ventricular hypertrophy can result in large R waves in V5–V6 and large S waves in V1–V2. The PR interval is lengthened in 1st degree heart block and shortened in Wolff-Parkinson-White. Atrial fibrillation will show absent P waves on a ragged baseline. T waves will be peaked in hyperkalaemia, and inverted in bundle branch block, ischaemia and ventricular hypertrophy. The QT interval will be lengthened in hypocalcaemia and shortened with increased calcium levels.

MULTIPLE BEST ANSWER QUESTIONS

1. Mediterranean diet   Answers: B C
A Mediterranean diet consists of fruit, fish, vegetables and poultry. It appears to decrease coronary artery disease more than the reduction achieved by a low fat diet.

2. Exercise   Answers: A C D
Regular exercise lowers blood pressure, and decreases risk of cancer of the colon, depression, and diabetes. Co-ordination is improved and the elderly may particularly benefit.

3. Cardiac rehabilitation after MI   Answers: A C D
Cardiac rehabilitation is offered to a limited number of patients after MI, and is usually carried out in hospitals, but can be carried out in General Practice if supported by a large team. It does not require a psychologist, though their input can be useful. Rehabilitation always has to include advice on diet and exercise and compliance with medication is essential.

4. Heart failure   Answers: B D E
Thiazides and Digoxin are used in treatment of heart failure but have not been shown to reduce mortality in randomised controlled trials.

5. Lipid lowering drugs   Answers: A B E
Post MI, the intention is to bring the cholesterol level below 5, but lipid lowering drugs are not currently recommended for primary prevention, unless the risk is >30%. Hypertension with no other risk factors would not require treatment at this level of cholesterol. They can be used in diabetes and compliance is a problem in some patients.

6. Hypertensive patients   Answers: A C
Thiazide diuretics are contraindicated in patients with glucose intolerance, but not calcium antagonists. Thiazide diuretics should be avoided in patients with gout. Beta-blockers should be avoided with obstructive airways disease.

7. Myocardial infarction   Answers: A C D
Following myocardial infarction (MI) ventricular fibrillation is most likely to occur within the first few hours and is one of the more easily correctable causes of early death. The ECG can remain normal following even an extensive MI. Thrombolytic therapy, when indicated, should be started early and is not dependent on resolution of chest pain.

8. Angina pectoris   Answers: A E
Angina with normal coronary arteries is found in cardiomyopathies, severe aortic stenosis and pulmonary hypertension, as well as in otherwise normal hearts when

coronary artery spasm or coronary blood flow abnormalities are implicated. The resting ECG is normal in 50% or more of patients between attacks. Many patients have angina on getting up in the morning and become symptom-free later in the day. ST segment elevation during an attack is unusual but may occur in 'variant' angina. The mechanism of angina on lying down is unknown but this symptom usually indicates severe coronary disease.

9.   Deep venous thrombosis   **Answers: B C D**
The most common cause of DVT is major surgery, especially after the age of 40. Long distance travel does cause DVT and several cases have been reported. It is best to stop combined contraceptive pill four weeks before major surgery. Calf vein thrombosis can be treated using compression bandages alone. Varicose veins have been shown to be a risk factor.

SINGLE BEST ANSWER QUESTIONS

1.   Hypertension   **Answer: D**
The therapeutic target for diabetics is much lower and thiazides can be used as first-line treatment in diabetes but not in patients with gout. Isolated systolic hypertension should be treated. Only about 33% of patients can be managed on monotherapy.

2.   Myocardial infarction   **Answer: A**
Age is an important factor in deciding the outcome of an infarct. Low blood pressure is a poor prognostic feature in the post-infarction phase. High heart rate on admission to hospital, anterior infarction pattern on ECG and previous myocardial infarction are poor prognostic indicators.

3.   Angioplasty   **Answer: E**
The left main stem is not suitable for angioplasty because occlusion during attempted angioplasty might be catastrophic. Multiple vessel angioplasty is now commonplace. Previous bypass surgery is not a contraindication to angioplasty, which may offer fewer risks than repeat surgery. The treatment of unstable angina may account for 25–30% of procedures in some centres.

DERMATOLOGY/ ENT PROBLEMS/ OPHTHALMOLOGY

DERMATOLOGY

EXTENDED MATCHING QUESTIONS

THEME: RASHES

1. **A** Dermatitis artefacta
2. **C** Lichen simplex
3. **B** Dermatitis herpetiformis
4. **D** Nodular prurigo

Suspect dermatitis artefacta if there are straight sides to the rash. Lichen simplex will heal if scratching is stopped. Nodular prurigo is one of the causes of rashes on the hands.

THEME: CAUSES OF NAIL DISCOLORATION

5. **F** Yellow nail syndrome
6. **C** Penicillamine
7. **A** Chloroquine
8. **B** Leuconychia
9. **E** Trauma
10. **D** Tinea infection
11. **B** Leuconychia

Penicillamine may stain the nails yellow, whereas chloroquine may stain the nails a blue-grey colour. Following trauma, often of a minor nature, the nails often have white streaks. Leuconychia is said to be inherited as an autosomal dominant gene; the whole nail becomes white. Tineal infection can cause yellow thickened areas of the nails with slow growth. In yellow nail syndrome the nail is curved longitudinally and transversally; there is an association with lymphoedema.

THEME: RASHES

12. **C** Infected eczema
13. **B** Ichthyosis
14. **A** Erythema multiforme
15. **D** Pustular psoriasis
16. **E** Scabies

With scabies, you will need to look carefully for burrows on the sides of the fingers. The lesions of pustular psoriasis are often seen on the soles of the feet and palms of the hand. Ichthyosis will cause scaly dry skin on the fingers. Erythema multiforme characteristically is seen as a large vesicle with a surrounding red halo. Infected eczema often has secondary staphylococcal infection.

THEME: SKIN CONDITIONS

17. **C** Guttate psoriasis
18. **B** Irritant contact dermatitis
19. **F** Pompholyx
20. **I** Erythrodermic psoriasis
21. **H** Asteatotic eczema

Irritant contact dermatitis differs from allergic contact dermatitis in that the area affected corresponds to the area of exposure. Allergic contact dermatitis tends to be progressively severe with repeated exposure and may cause irritation at distant sites, e.g. earrings and watches in the case of nickel sensitivity. Psoriasis is generally diagnosable by its characteristic lesions, which show pinpoint bleeding when removed.

THEME: LEG ULCERS

22. **B** Venous ulcers
23. **B** Venous ulcers
24. **A** Ischaemic ulcers
25. **A** Ischaemic ulcers
26. **B** Venous ulcers

It is important to be able to distinguish venous and arterial leg ulcers. Venous ulcers are painless, pigmented, and there is usually oedema and induration with eczematous skin surrounding the ulcer. Ischaemic leg ulcers tend to be punched out and necrotic; they are frequently painful.

MULTIPLE BEST ANSWER QUESTIONS

1. Nails   Answers: A B C
Decreased nutritional supply to the nail matrix can lead to defective nail formation, resulting in a transverse groove made of thinner nail plate. Since fingernails grow at about 1 mm/week it is possible to date previous illnesses. The other major cause of these grooves is psoriasis. Opacity of the nail is suggestive of diabetes mellitus, cardiac failure and psoriasis. Blue nails are found as a side-effect of anti-malarial drugs such as chloroquine; whereas green nails are caused by Pseudomonas *spp*. Splinter haemorrhages are seen in bacterial endocarditis. Longitudinal ridges can be seen in lichen planus.

2. Pregnancy   Answers: B D
The condition of most patients with atopic eczema improves during pregnancy. However some patients suffer deterioration which may be caused by increased excoriation from pruritus gravidarum. Hidradenitis suppurativa also usually improves during pregnancy.

3. Drug reactions   Answers: B E
Oral contraceptives are characteristically linked with melasma, a brownish pigmentation on the face. Both codeine and aspirin can cause urticaria. Exfoliative dermatitis is usually caused by carbamazepine, allopurinol, gold, phenytoin, captopril or diltiazem but not tetracycline. Fucidin usually causes eczema rather than pigmentation.

4. Granuloma annulare   Answers: C D E
Granuloma annulare is a disease of unknown aetiology which often starts in a single area but may develop into multiple lesions. It is usually confined to the extremities and is painless. The disease may persist for many years and there is no effective treatment. There is a probable association with diabetes mellitus.

5. Erythema nodosum   Answers: B C
Herpes simplex is usually associated with erythema multiforme. Hyperthyroidism usually causes pruritus or urticaria rather than erythema nodosum. The infections associated with erythema nodosum include tuberculosis and leprosy. Inflammatory bowel disease and many rheumatic diseases are associated with erythema nodosum.

6. Drugs that exacerbate psoriasis   Answers: A D
Lithium and beta-blockers can precipitate and exacerbate psoriasis. Hydralazine has been linked with a number of conditions, for example, systemic lupus erythematosus, but not psoriasis.

7.   Alopecia areata   Answers: B D E
Hair loss in alopecia areata may occur at any site. Most of the follicles retain the
ability to form new hairs. Alopecia areata may be associated with frank or
subclinical auto-immune thyroid disease and with Down's syndrome. Nail pitting or
roughness is commonly found in alopecia areata.

8.   Acne vulgaris   Answers: A B C
In 60% of teenagers acne will be of sufficient severity for them to treat themselves
with proprietary preparations or seek medical advice. Circulating levels of androgen
are usually normal in patients with acne. The blackhead is caused by the plug within
the pilosebaceous duct expanding to dilate the pilosebaceous orifice and gradually
become extruded. The severity of acne is directly related to the degree of secretion
of sebum.

SINGLE BEST ANSWER QUESTIONS

1.   Basal cell carcinoma   Answer: A
Basal cell carcinoma (BCC) is the most common skin malignancy in Caucasians.
Basal cell carcinoma sometimes occurs on covered skin sites. Curettage and cautery
in skilled hands remains a perfectly acceptable means of treatment.

2.   Multiple seborrhoeic warts   Answer: A
Seborrhoeic warts may occur in any area where there are pilo-sebaceous follicles,
but they are seen predominantly on the face and trunk. They are non-infective.
They are best removed by curettage or cryotherapy.

3.   Erythema nodosum   Answer: A
Erythema nodosum may be due to an underlying systemic disease e.g. Crohn's
disease, ulcerative colitis or sarcoidosis. It can be caused by various drugs, notably
sulphonamides and oral contraceptives, and by preceding infection, especially
streptococcal.

4.   Molluscum contagiosum   Answer: A
A review in the BMJ in 1999 found that scarring was most common after phenol
ablation. Furthermore there was no evidence to support any of the treatments over
watchful waiting. The condition is most commonly seen in children but is also seen
in HIV positive patients. The average duration for the condition is 8 months.

5.   Venous leg ulcers   Answer: B
Only compression bandaging has been shown to be effective. Hyperbaric oxygen is
a treatment for radio-osteonecrosis. The key to safe and effective treatment of
venous ulcers is measurement of the ankle:brachial blood pressure index to avoid
inadvertent treatment of arterial ulcers.

ENT PROBLEMS

EXTENDED MATCHING QUESTIONS

THEME: LESIONS ON THE EAR

1. **A** Chilblains
2. **E** Squamous cell cancer
3. **F** Tophi
4. **B** Kerato-acanthoma
5. **D** Rodent ulcer
6. **C** Psoriatic

Chilblains are common, painful and itchy. Squamous cell cancer lesions of the ear are slow growing lesions found on the helix. Tophi in the ear are usually found on the antihelix. Kerato-acanthoma lesions are rapidly growing and are also usually found on the helix. Rodent ulcer ear lesions are usually found behind and below the ear. Psoriatic lesions are found in the external auditory meatus and on the skin behind and below the ear.

THEME: HOARSENES

7. **D** Pharyngeal neoplasia
8. **E** Smoking
9. **C** Myxoedema
10. **D** Pharyngeal neoplasia
11. **B** Gastro-oesophageal reflux

Hoarseness is an abnormality of the voice. If associated with weight loss, consider upper or lower respiratory tract cancer. Smoking causes trauma to the larynx. Associated dysphagia is suggestive of upper respiratory cancer and palsies of the larynx or pharynx. Long-standing myxoedema is associated with a hoarse voice.

THEME: EARACHE

12. **I** Ramsay Hunt syndrome
13. **D** Glue ear
14. **J** Cerebellopontine angle tumours
15. **A** Otitis media
16. **B** Otitis externa

Ramsay Hunt syndrome, herpes zoster oticus, is treated with aciclovir. It may be associated with facial nerve palsy. Acoustic neuromas may be misdiagnosed as Menière's and should be suspected, particularly in patients with unilateral sensorineural deafness. Viral otitis media commonly causes a febrile illness in children with few localizing symptoms. Examination should always include the ears, nose and throat. Otitis externa may be secondary to minor ear trauma, middle ear disease or caused by repeated immersion e.g. in surfers and swimmers.

MULTIPLE BEST ANSWER QUESTIONS

1.   Glue ear   **Answers: A E**
Atopic children have increased incidence and episodes tend to be more prolonged; bottle-fed babies have greater incidence of atopy. Children with facial anomalies are more prone to glue ear due to poor drainage. Neomycin and meningitis cause sensorineural deafness.

2.   Oral cancer   **Answers: A B E**
Several studies have shown an association between high alcohol consumption and oral cancer. Iron deficiency, but not folate deficiency, predisposes to oral cancer. Cigar smoking is associated with leukoplakia of the floor of the mouth in women.

3.   Otitis externa   **Answers: A C D**
Any local trauma (e.g. poking the ears, foreign body in ear) will pre-dispose to otitis externa. Certain occupations such as mining and diving have increased incidence of otitis externa. Usually otitis media is more common in the under 5-year-olds. Psoriasis as well as eczema and seborrhoeic dermatitis are pre-disposing factors.

4.   Drugs causing dry mouth   **Answers: B D E**
Antihistamines, phenothiazines and amphetamines can cause a dry mouth. Tricyclic but not monoamine oxidase inhibitor antidepressants cause a dry mouth, as do bronchodilators but not bronchoconstrictors.

SINGLE BEST ANSWER QUESTIONS

1.   Conductive deafness   **Answer: A**
Post-meningitis, congenital rubella and kernicterus cause sensorineural deafness rather than conductive deafness, which is caused by glue ear, large perforations and destructions, dislocation or adhesion of the ossicles.

2.   Mild allergic rhinitis   **Answer: B**
The best initial treatment for mild allergic rhinitis is an oral non-sedating antihistamine. Chronic nasal blockage may require the use of nasal steroids. Regular use of xylometolazone may cause rhinitis medicamentosa, a paradoxical increase in rhinitis. RAST testing is unnecessary unless a specific trigger is suspected or symptoms are particularly severe. Reduction in house dust mite exposure has not been shown to significantly reduce symptoms.

3.   Sensorineural deafness   **Answer: D**
The commonest cause of isolated sensorineural deafness in this age group is
presbyacusis. In Menière's disease, symptoms of tinnitus, vertigo and a fullness are
common. Infections such as measles and mumps, or ototoxic medications would
usually present earlier. Barotrauma and otosclerosis are causes of conductive
deafness.

OPHTHALMOLOGY

EXTENDED MATCHING QUESTIONS

THEME: SUDDEN LOSS OF VISION

1. **C** Optic neuritis
2. **D** Senile macular degeneration
3. **E** Toxic optic neuropathy
4. **B** Migraine
5. **A** Central retinal vein occlusion

In the sudden loss of vision associated with migraine, there is a complete recovery from the loss of vision which often, but not always, occurs with headache. In central retinal vein occlusion, the visual loss develops over a few hours. There is extensive haemorrhage visible at the fundus.

Senile macular degeneration is a gradually progressive loss of vision in an older person. There is preservation of peripheral fields. Optic neuritis is a gradual loss of vision in people between 20 and 45 years old. The peripheral vision is intact. Toxic optic neuropathy tends to occur in heavy cigarette smokers. Peripheral vision remains largely intact.

THEME: RED EYE

6. **D** Keratitis
7. **B** Episcleritis
8. **C** Iritis
9. **A** Acute glaucoma
10. **E** Sub-conjunctival haemorrhage

In the red eye caused by episcleritis, there is slight or no pain. Vision tends to be normal and the red eye will settle without treatment. Sub-conjunctival haemorrhage is painless and vision is normal. Keratitis is associated with impaired vision. An ulcer may be found near the visual axis. Acute glaucoma is accompanied by severe pain with severe visual impairment. Vomiting commonly occurs. In iritis, the pupil is small and often distorted.

THEME: VISUAL FIELD DEFECTS

11. **A** Arcuate scotoma
12. **C** Centrocaecal scotoma
13. **D** Ring scotoma
14. **B** Central scotoma

Visual field defects can be important in localising and defining a disease process. A central scotoma is characteristic of disease affecting the macula, whereas toxic neuropathy can produce a centrocaecal scotoma. A ring scotoma is typical of the field defect in retinitis pigmentosa, while an arcuate scotoma is characteristic of glaucoma.

THEME: EYE LESIONS

15. **D** Pterygium
16. **A** Corneal arcus
17. **E** Sub-conjunctival haemorrhage
18. **B** Kayser-Fleischer rings
19. **C** Pinguecula
20. **B** Kayser-Fleischer rings
21. **E** Sub-conjunctival haemorrhage

Pingueculae and pterygia are both found between the canthus and the corneal edge. A pterygium is a triangular fold of conjunctiva, whereas a pinguecula is a yellow deposit beneath the conjunctiva. A corneal arcus is very common and is a white ring near the outer margin of the cornea. Kayser-Fleischer rings are very rare, occurring in Wilson's disease as a deposit of copper at the periphery of the cornea. Sub-conjunctival haemorrhages are very common; they are bright red marks resulting spontaneously or from prolonged forceful coughing or straining.

MULTIPLE BEST ANSWER QUESTIONS

1. Acute iritis   **Answers: B C**

Acute iritis causes blurred vision with photophobia and small pupil. Needs to be referred at once since it is a threat to sight. Purulent discharge usually signifies conjunctivitis, while a hard and tender eye suggests acute glaucoma.

2. Visual problems in myopia   **Answers: A D**

When conducting ophthalmoscopy in a patient with myopia, the minus lenses will be needed. The disc may look large and pale and there may be surrounding chorioretinal atrophy.

3. Visual fundus findings   **Answers: B D F G**

Hard exudates are caused by lipoprotein leaking out of blood vessels and are noted in diabetes and hypertension. They are well defined yellow-white deposits often in rings.

Soft exudates look like deposits of cotton wool. They occur in infarcted retina, often being associated with features of retinal ischaemia such as new vessel formation and venous dilatation. Soft exudates are due to the swelling of the axons in the nerve fibre layer of the retina.

SINGLE BEST ANSWER QUESTIONS

1.   Causes of blindness   **Answer: D**
Macular degeneration accounts for over one-third of those blind over the age of 65 years.

2.   Causes of blindness   **Answer: A**
Diabetic retinopathy causes about 20% of the blindness in patients in the age range 45–64 years.

3.   Cataracts   **Answer: B**
In many cases, cataracts are age-related, appearing first when a person is in his or her 40s or 50s, but not affecting vision until after age 60. Other causes of cataracts include injury to the eye, untreated eye inflammation, diabetes, drugs (such as cortisone), exposure to X-rays and ultraviolet (UV) light and heredity. Congenital cataracts may occur as a result of an infection that happened during pregnancy, especially toxoplasmosis, cytomegalovirus, syphilis, rubella or herpes simplex. In infants and young children, cataracts may also be one symptom of a metabolic disease affecting the body's processing of carbohydrates, amino acids, calcium or copper. Myotonic dystrophy is associated with early cataracts.

4.   Diabetic maculopathy   **Answer: A**
Maculopathy as opposed to retinopathy is certainly more common in the older patient with NIDDM. The patient may be registered blind because of the damage to the very sensitive macular area. However, even though the patient may be unable to read, they may retain excellent peripheral vision. Treatment of maculopathy is usually with small, focal laser burns to the macular area, avoiding the fovea. This is in contrast to treatment for proliferative retinopathy which usually involves several thousand burns to the peripheral retina. Drusen are a normal feature in some patients. Hard exudates, often in rings, are characteristic of diabetic maculopathy. Painful visual loss is not a feature of maculopathy and would suggest glaucoma, uveitis or another lesion.

5.   Anterior uveitis   **Answer: B**
Blurring of vision, small pupil and photophobia suggest anterior uveitis. Other causes of 'red-eye' are subconjunctival haemorrhage, which is not painful, and acute closed-angle glaucoma and keratitis which are painful.

ENDOCRINOLOGY/ METABOLIC

EXTENDED MATCHING QUESTIONS

THEME: ENDOCRINE DISEASES

1. **A** Acromegaly
2. **D** Diabetes insipidus
3. **C** Cushing's
4. **B** Conn's
5. **E** Simmond's

Cushing's disease and syndrome are associated with excess corticosteroids. Conn's disease is caused by excess aldosterone. Diabetes insipidus is due to a deficiency of ADH. Acromegaly is caused by excess growth hormone. Simmond's disease is associated with deficiencies of GH, FSH and LH.

THEME: METABOLIC BONE DISEASE

6. **E** Paget's
7. **G** Rickets
8. **C** Osteomalacia
9. **B** Hypoparathyroidism
10. **E** Paget's
11. **A** Hyperparathyroidism
12. **G** Rickets
13. **D** Osteoporosis

You need a good knowledge of General Medicine for some questions. Osteoporosis is common and its prevention is a major reason for prescribing HRT. Osteomalacia often presents with bone pain and tenderness and is associated with moderately increased alkaline phosphatase, and decreased calcium and phosphate. Rickets is seen in children and can present with leg and chest deformities. Paget's disease is associated with a hugely increased alkaline phosphatase. It presents as bone pain and tenderness, with bone deformity. The sacrum and lumbar spine are the most commonly affected bones. Paget's can be complicated by progressive occlusion of skull foramina causing deafness, and also by high output cardiac failure. Hyperparathyroidism is associated with increased calcium levels, bone cysts and sub-periosteal erosions in the phalanges. However, hypoparathyroidism is associated with decreased calcium levels but increased phosphate levels, with calcification sometimes seen in the basal ganglia.

THEME: ARTHRITIS

14. **H** Ankylosing spondylitis
15. **I** Reiter's syndrome
16. **C** Psoriatic arthritis
17. **E** Septic arthritis
18. **G** Gout
19. **L** Rubella

Features strongly suggestive of inflammatory spinal disease are insidious onset, onset before 40 years of age, early morning stiffness and improvement with exercise. With suitable treatment prognosis is excellent. There is a 50% chance of passing the HLA B27 gene to offspring and a 33% chance of developing disease if HLA B27 positive. Reiter's may start after gastrointestinal infection or urogenital infection. The classical triad of arthritis, conjunctivitis and urethritis is often incomplete. It may be associated with the characteristic skin lesion keratoderma blenorrhagica. In psoriatic arthropathy the joint activity tends to match the plaque activity. Where nail disease is present, small joint involvement is likely. Septic arthritis usually infects a single joint with pain, fever, erythema and swelling. Gonococcal arthritis is common in women and homosexual men and usually occurs within 3 weeks of infection. Treatment is with benzylpenicillin. Trauma, surgery, drugs, alcohol or starvation may cause gout. Pseudogout is the deposition of calcium pyrophosphate, typically in the knees. Rubella may cause an acute arthritis similar to rubella, with a positive rheumatoid factor. A self-limiting arthralgia may also be seen with rubella vaccination.

MULTIPLE BEST ANSWER QUESTIONS

1.   Gout   Answers: A B E
The annual incidence of gout in the UK is about 1 in 3000 population. The reason for the male predominance is not known. Two types of people are particularly affected: obese, male heavy drinkers of alcohol and elderly patients taking thiazide diuretics.

2.   Features of osteoporosis   Answers: B C D
The WHO defines osteopenia as a bone density one standard deviation below the mean, with osteoporosis being a bone density of greater than 2.5 standard deviations below the mean.

More than 30% of women and more than 10% of men will have an osteoporotic fracture during their lives. Bone densitometry is usually maximal at the early adult stage beginning to fall at about 40. It can predict risk but cannot identify those who will sustain a fracture.

3.   Wilson's disease   Answers: D E
Wilson's disease is inherited as an autosomal recessive disorder of copper metabolism, due to an absence of a copper binding globulin. Symptoms appear in early adult life with copper deposited in the liver, basal ganglia, cerebrum, renal tubules and eyes, producing Kayser Fleischer rings.

4.   Non-insulin dependent diabetes (NIDDM)   Answers: A D
Although insulin resistance is a major problem in the obese non-insulin dependent diabetic, patients presenting with hyperosmolar coma are typically very sensitive to insulin. The half-life of glibenclamide is relatively short, but it has active metabolites with a long half-life. Glipizide and its metabolites have a short duration of action and are therefore much safer in the elderly. Metformin does not normally induce clinical hypoglycaemia, even in overdose. Facial flushing with alcohol occurs in some patients treated with chlorpropamide.

5.   Hyperuricaemia   Answers: A B D
Hyperuricaemia is induced by frusemide (also with thiazides) and polycythaemia rubra vera (due to increased purine turnover). Multiple myeloma is associated with hyperuricaemia due to increased purine turnover but also treatment with anti-metabolites causes tissue destruction and a further rise of serum uric acid. There is no such association with diabetes nor myxoedema.

6.   Risk factors for osteoporosis   Answers: A B
Causes of osteoporosis include genetic factors (60%), lack of exercise, low dietary calcium, cigarette smoking, excessive alcohol consumption, amenorrhoea, vitamin D deficiency, low body weight and early menopause. All *accelerate* the rate at which bone is lost. The other causes include oral corticosteroids, hyperthyroidism, hypogonadism, rheumatoid arthritis and immobilisation of joints.

7.   Haemochromatosis   Answers: C D E
Haemochromatosis is inherited as an autosomal dominant and results in excess iron absorption and deposition in the liver, pancreas, heart, synovial membranes and endocrine glands. It is seen mainly in men over 30 years old. It may present with diabetes, with skin pigmentation (due to melanin), with hepatomegaly, polyarthropathy, or cardiac problems. Wilson's disease is a disorder of copper metabolism, which may result in Kayser Fleischer rings in the eyes.

8.   Hypoglycaemia   Answers: B C D
Alcoholics who do not eat may develop fasting hypoglycaemia due to depletion of glycogen stores by starvation and inhibition of hepatic gluconeogenesis. Other causes include hypopituitarism, Addison's disease, Von Gierke's disease, insulinomas, overtreatment with insulin and severe liver disease. Hepatic carcinomas, mesotheliomas or retroperitoneal fibrosarcomas may cause hypoglycaemia due to secretion of a pro-insulin-like peptide.

9.   Pregnancies of diabetic women   Answers: B C E

Diabetic women usually have hydramnios and there is an increased incidence of pre-eclampsia. There is a four-fold increase in congenital abnormalities. Babies born to diabetic women are usually large since insulin has a growth hormone-like effect in the fetus. The exact cause of increased intra-uterine deaths is unknown.

SINGLE BEST ANSWER QUESTIONS

1.   Hypothyroidism   Answer: B

In a thyroid gland that is failing, the serum T_3 level may remain in the normal range although the serum T_4 level is reduced and serum TSH level elevated. Eventually the serum T_3 level may also fall into the subnormal range. Infiltration of subcutaneous tissues with mucopolysaccharides causes typical facial puffiness, ankle swelling and carpal tunnel syndrome, the last by compression of the median nerve within the flexor retinaculum of the wrist. Pretibial myxoedema is a feature of Graves' disease. The macrocytosis occurs in isolation but there is a high incidence of pernicious anaemia in patients with primary hypothyroidism. However, menorrhagia or defective absorption of iron (resulting from achlorhydria) may lead to a microcytic hypochromic anaemia.

2.   Carpal tunnel syndrome   Answer: C

In carpal tunnel syndrome, the median nerve may be compressed by changes in the wrist joint (rheumatoid arthritis, acromegaly), soft tissue swelling (myxoedema) or fluid retention (pregnancy). Symptoms are usually worse after a night's rest and improve as activity mobilises extra-cellular fluid

GASTROENTEROLOGY/ NUTRITION

EXTENDED MATCHING QUESTIONS

THEME: CAUSES OF ABDOMINAL PAIN

1. **E** Pancreatitis
2. **C** Diverticular disease
3. **B** Irritable bowel syndrome
4. **D** Ischaemic colitis
5. **B** Irritable bowel syndrome
6. **F** Cholecystitis
7. **A** Crohn's disease

With clinical scenarios, read the scenario and think about the likely diagnosis in ordinary clinical practice. There will be pointers towards the correct option. Read these scenarios again with the 'correct' answers in mind. In these scenarios, consider the angina and bloody diarrhoea in a 69-year-old as significant and the diagnosis of ischaemic colitis becomes obvious. Similarly, the anal tags and generalised abdominal tenderness point towards Crohn's disease.

THEME: CHANGE IN BOWEL HABIT

8. **A** Toddler diarrhoea
9. **J** Irritable bowel syndrome
10. **C** Ulcerative colitis
11. **H** Carcinoid syndrome
12. **K** Hyperthyroidism
13. **G** Coeliac disease
14. **I** Giardiasis

Irritable bowel is sometimes considered a diagnosis of exclusion; however, diagnostic criteria (Rome and Manning) exist. Patients with ulcerative colitis usually experience symptoms for the first time in their 20s. Long-term surveillance is necessary due to late malignant change. Carcinoid also often produces sharp right hypochondrial pain due to hepatomegaly. Classically, coeliac disease presents as failure to thrive in children. Recently evidence of coeliac disease has been found in patients presenting to their GPs with vague non-specific symptoms of lethargy and malaise. Giardia may be seen not only in travellers but also in gay men, where it is sexually transmitted, in some patients it may cause malabsorption.

THEME: INDIGESTION

15. **C** Alginates
16. **B** Proton pump inhibitor
17. **H** Misoprostol
18. **D** Nissan's fundoplication
19. **A** H_2 receptor antagonist

Reflux is common in pregnancy due to progesterone-mediated relaxation of the lower oesophageal sphincter. Alginates such as Gaviscon are usually sufficient. In the treatment of reflux, mild symptoms should be treated with H_2RAs or alginates, those with proven erosive oesophagitis should be treated with PPIs at an initial healing dose then at a lower doses until a maintenance level is reached. *Helicobacter pylori* treatment is indicated for dyspepsia, not reflux.

MULTIPLE BEST ANSWER QUESTIONS

1. Gallstones   **Answers: B E**
The incidence of stones in the gall bladder rises with age. Many stones remain asymptomatic. Pigment, rather than cholesterol, stones are associated with bacteria in the bile. Chenodeoxycholic acid is ineffective for pigment stones. Cholecystectomy remains the standard treatment for symptomatic gallstones.

2. *Helicobacter pylori*   **Answers: A B**
Helicobacter pylori infection is usually acquired in the first five years of life. The infection is found in about 50% of people over 50, but the rate of infection is decreasing with improve socio-economic conditions. Infection is associated with duodenal and gastric ulcer, and also gastric carcinoma. Blood tests for *H. pylori* can be confusing since antibodies remain present, but the breath test becomes negative once *H. pylori* is eradicated.

3. Acute gastroenteritis   **Answers: A B**
Gastroenteritis in at risk groups, such as infants and elderly patients, produces dehydration. Oral rehydration therapy (ORT) corrects the dehydration. Commercial preparations are adequate for the treatment of mild or moderate dehydration commonly seen in the UK. Food has little or no effect on the diarrhoea and should be encouraged as soon as practicable. Antibiotics are rarely required but erythromycin may be needed for Campylobacter infection with systemic upset.

4. Crohn's disease   **Answers: A B**
Crohn's is a chronic inflammatory disease affecting any part of the gut from the mouth to the anus. It is a trans-mural inflammation with 'skip lesions' (normal bowel segments). Complications include strictures, fistulae and malabsorption. Anaemia is from malabsorption and loss of blood or protein into bowel. Thrombophlebitis is usually noted with ulcerative colitis.

5.   Peptic ulceration   Answers: A E

The association with *H. pylori* infection is well proven and endoscopy is useful, but not an essential investigation. Having milk or food normally relieves pain associated with duodenal ulcer, and vomiting is present only with obstruction. Although proton pump inhibitors are now widely used H_2-antagonists still have a place.

6.   Duodenal ulceration   Answers: A B

There is no evidence to prove a causal relationship between non-steroidal anti-inflammatory drugs and duodenal ulceration. Duodenal ulceration is often a chronic disease with frequent relapses. Duodenal ulceration causes epigastric pain some hours after a meal, when the patient is hungry.

7.   Cancer of the colon   Answers: B C D

Early diagnosis is important in cancer of the colon. At present the overall 5-year survival is only 35%. Patients at particular risk of developing cancer of the colon include those with inflammatory bowel disease and patients with a family history of polyposis coli. Patients with a family history of either colonic cancer diagnosed before the age of 45 years or with two first degree relatives with cancer of the colon are also at increased risk. Screening for faecal occult blood depends on a tumour bleeding which may occur late in the disease. The test has a low sensitivity and specificity.

8.   Diverticular disease of the colon   Answers: A B D

High fibre diet prevents diverticular disease of the colon. The majority of patients are asymptomatic and do not present to General Practitioners, when symptomatic high fibre diet is usually prescribed. Acute diverticulitis is a rare complication, approximately 1%.

9.   Colorectal cancer   Answers: D E

Change in bowel habit can be a feature, but does not need urgent referral, and bleeding with anal symptoms and lower abdominal pain are possible symptoms, but again not requiring urgent referral. Hb <11g/dl in men and abdominal mass do require urgent referral.

SINGLE BEST ANSWER QUESTIONS

1.   Duodenal ulcer   Answer: A

Studies have shown no difference in healing rates with ranitidine or cimetidine using single or divided daily doses. Failure to heal is often due to poor compliance. Recurrence may be entirely asymptomatic. You should be aware of the link between *Helicobacter pylori* and gastroduodenal disease, and choice of therapy. Many people are infected with *H. pylori* and more than half the population over the age of 50 have evidence of gastritis. However, in the absence of peptic ulceration, you should not try to eradicate the organism.

Most *H. pylori* eradication regimes are based on a proton pump inhibitor or H_2 receptor antagonist, plus one or more antibiotics. Triple therapy involving the use of two antibiotics is more effective in eradication than dual pathology.

2.   Jaundice   Answer: C

Jaundice from liver damage is caused by paracetamol, halothane and isoniazid. Arsenic causes fibrosis. Methyldopa interferes with the normal bilirubin pathway. Cholestasis occurs with chlorpromazine and the oral contraceptive pill; the latter can also cause hepatic vein occlusion.

3.   Examination of biliary system   Answer: A

Oral cholecystography and biliary ultrasound are similar in terms of specificity and sensitivity. The cause of bile duct obstruction can be demonstrated in the majority of cases. However in about 5% of obstructive jaundice cases the bile ducts are not dilated at the time of examination, especially if the jaundice is not severe or is of short duration. Space-occupying lesions of the liver of about 2cm in diameter and occasionally 1cm can be visualised. Metastases, primary liver cancer, cysts or abscesses can be identified. Ultrasonography also demonstrates ascites.

4.   Irritable bowel syndrome   Answer: A

A significant minority of patients relate their symptoms, usually of painless diarrhoea, to an episode of infective diarrhoea often contracted abroad. The whole gut may be involved and gastric symptoms may coexist with colonic ones. A barium enema on colonoscopy is not essential in most patients especially when all the typical features are present in the young person. The diagnosis is common in the elderly but more extensive investigations are required to rule out alternative diagnoses. Despite the similarities between the irritable bowel syndrome and diverticular disease evidence is lacking that the irritable bowel syndrome precedes the diverticular disease in individuals.

5.   Drugs causing constipation   Answer: D

Aluminium trisilicate, tricyclic antidepressants and oral contraceptives may cause constipation. Iron most commonly causes constipation but it can also cause diarrhoea. Cimetidine causes diarrhoea rather than constipation.

6.   Irritable bowel syndrome   Answer: A

Irritable bowel syndrome (IBS) most commonly presents in the mid 30s: patients are seldom over 50 years. Symptoms of ibs are common in childhood and many adults with IBS give a history which extends back to childhood.

7.   Diverticular disease   Answer: D

Diverticular disease is the clinical syndrome which complicates diverticulosis, so by definition it cannot occur without symptoms. The sigmoid colon is the most common segment of the bowel to be affected by diverticular disease. Rectal bleeding seldom occurs, but when it does it usually settles spontaneously without treatment. The treatment for acute diverticular disease is hospitalisation, rest, analgesia (avoiding morphine) and antibiotics including metronidazole. Surgery is rarely necessary acutely.

INFECTIOUS DISEASES/ HAEMATOLOGY/ IMMUNOLOGY/ ALLERGIES/GENETICS

EXTENDED MATCHING QUESTIONS

THEME: CHROMOSOME DISORDERS

1. **C** X-linked
2. **A** Autosomal Dominant
3. **B** Autosomal Recessive
4. **C** X-linked
5. **A** Autosomal Dominant

Haemophilia (A and B) is a sex-linked disease, as is red-green colour blindness. These problems will therefore only rarely (but not never) be seen in females. Familial hypercholesterolaemia is one of the commonest inherited disorders in the Western World, and is autosomal dominant. Familial adenomatous polyposis coli is uncommon, accounting for about 1% of all colon cancers. It is inherited as an autosomal dominant. Cystic fibrosis is one of the commonest autosomal recessive conditions.

THEME: INFECTIVE AGENTS ASSOCIATED WITH TUMOURS

6. **B** *Helicobacter pylori*
7. **C** Hepatitis B virus
8. **D** Human herpes virus type 8
9. **E** Human papillomavirus
10. **E** Human papillomavirus

Primary gastric lymphoma is strongly associated with *Helicobacter pylori* infection. The development of hepatocellular carcinoma is linked with the Hepatitis B virus. Kaposi's sarcoma is common in patients with AIDS and there is a firm association with Human herpes virus type 8.

All warts are benign tumours and caused by Human papillomavirus (HPV). Genital warts are caused by HPV types 6 and 11.

Other HPV serotypes, expecially 16 and 18, have been implicated in the development of cervical intraepithelial neoplasia and invasive cervical cancer.

MULTIPLE BEST ANSWER QUESTIONS

1.   Turner's syndrome   Answers: A B
Turner's syndrome (XO genotype) is frequently associated with coarctation of the
aorta, streak gonads, primary amenorrhoea and short stature. It is commonly seen in
spontaneous abortions. They have neck webbing and increased carrying angle at
the elbow.

2.   Pertussis immunisation   Answers: B D
Absolute contraindications to pertussis immunisation are:
- Severe general reactions. Fever equal to or more than 39.5°C within 48 hours of
  vaccine; anaphylaxis; generalised collapse; prolonged unresponsiveness; prolonged inconsolable screaming and convulsions occurring within 72 hours.
- Severe local reaction to the preceding dose. An area of extensive redness and
  swelling which becomes indurated and involves most of the antero-lateral area
  of the thigh or the major part of the circumference of the upper arm.
- Unstable neurological condition. Unlike symptomatic hypoglycaemic fits, the
  outcome of hypocalcaemic fits in the neonatal period is usually good and not
  associated with neuro-developmental problems.

3.   Autosomal dominant diseases   Answers: B D E
Down's syndrome is a trisomy 21 while cystic fibrosis is autosomal recessive
inheritance.

4.   Diarrhoea in a patient with AIDS   Answers: A B E
Any unusual organism isolated from the rectum should alert the clinician to the
diagnosis, but gonococcus, herpes simplex, *Giardia lamblia* and cytomegalovirus
may be found. A full range of investigations may be required for accurate diagnosis,
but will depend on the individual case. In particular, cytomegalovirus may only be
diagnosed by histological examination. Whilst all bodily fluids from AIDS patients
should be treated with caution, HIV has not been isolated from stools. However,
beware bloody diarrhoea. There have only been a small number of proven cases of
seroconversion from any source in health workers caring for infected patients.
Cryptosporidium can cause a severe diarrhoea which is often recurrent. It is often
difficult to treat but may respond to erythromycin.

5.   Infectious hepatitis   Answers: B C
Hepatitis C (previously called non A-non B Hepatitis) is now the commonest blood
borne hepatitis in the UK. Hepatitis D (Delta agent) co-exists with hepatitis B and is
relatively rare in the UK. Hepatitis E is food/water borne producing an illness similar
to hepatitis A. It is hoped the widespread vaccination against hepatitis B will greatly
reduce the incidence of primary hepatoma.

6. Glandular fever
Answers: A B E

In glandular fever, liver function tests are abnormal in over 80% but less than 10% are jaundiced. If given ampicillin, patients will develop a rash. The sore throat lasts for more than seven days. Patients can have prolonged lethargy and depression for many months after the acute illness. About 80% of patients have a positive monospot test. Antibody production may be slow and you may need to repeat the test in two weeks to confirm the diagnosis.

7. Normal iron metabolism
Answers: A C

The normal daily requirement for adults is 1–2 mg. Haemoglobin accounts for about 75% of total body iron. Haem iron, present in meat, is more readily absorbed than inorganic iron. Although inorganic iron usually predominates in the diet, relatively little can be made available for absorption, the exact amount depending on the presence or absence of dietary components and gastrointestinal secretions that enhance the solubility of iron. There is no physiological route for iron excretion.

8. Pneumococcal immunisation
Answers: A C

Pneumococcal immunisation should be considered for all those in whom pneumococcal infection is more common or more serious. This includes patients with homozygous sickle cell disease, asplenia and chronic renal, cardiac, liver or respiratory disease. In HIV positive patients, the serological response to vaccination, and hence benefit, declines with the increased immuno-compromised state. Routine revaccination is not normally recommended.

9. Pneumococcal infections
Answers: B D F

There is a need to consider pneumococcal vaccination in patients with post-splenectomy, multiple myeloma and sickle cell disease.

SINGLE BEST ANSWER QUESTIONS

1. Measles
Answer: B

The respiratory complications of measles include pneumonia, bronchiolitis and bronchiectasis but not recurrent pnumothoraces. Corneal ulceration may occur. Severe infection from prolonged and intense exposure to infected siblings in the same household is more likely to cause fatal disease than malnutrition. Lifelong immunity is established after natural infection.

2. Depressed immune response
Answer: A

Malnutrition rather than obesity may cause a depressed immune response. Extremes of life represent periods of increased risk from infection, for example, the elderly are particularly susceptible to pneumococcal pneumonia. Certain infections depress the immune response, as in AIDS.

3.   Red blood cell macrocytosis   Answer: B
The macrocytosis of coeliac disease is usually due to folate deficiency. Alcohol
makes the red cells large directly, through secondary folate deficiency and with liver
disease. In aplasia, younger larger red cells leave the bone marrow.

4.   HIV antibody test   Answer: D
General epidemiological data suggest that the interval between HIV exposure and
seroconversion is usually no more than 2 months, and this justifies setting a 3–6
month limit to the follow-up of individuals who have been sexually exposed to HIV
infection. Antibody status usually, but not always, indicates the ability of an
individual to infect other people; for example, there are several instances of HIV
transmission by blood donations from seronegative donors.
False-positive antibody tests are not uncommon so all positive results must be cross-
checked.

5.   Haematological conditions   Answer: D
Iron deficiency is linked with microcytic anaemia, as are vitamins A and C and
pyridoxine deficiencies. Cobalamin deficiency is linked with megaloblastic
anaemia, as is folic acid deficiency.

6.   Sickle cell anaemia   Answer: B
Folic acid deficiency may increase aplastic crises and folate supplements are
recommended, particularly during pregnancy when crisis frequency may increase.
There is chronic haemolysis which results in normal or raised serum iron levels.
Recurrent tissue infarcts lead to splenic fibrosis and shrinkage, pulmonary
hypertension and focal neurological signs. Recurrent haematuria, occasionally
nephrotic syndrome, aseptic femoral head necrosis and priapism may all occur.
Septic complications are most frequent and life threatening. Pneumococcal
septicaemia is a major hazard because of hyposplenism. Prophylactic penicillin and
immunisation are used.

7.   Complications of rheumatoid disease   Answer: A
Finger clubbing is not associated with rheumatoid disease but swan-neck
deformities of the fingers are recognised signs. The systemic manifestations include
pericarditis, pleurisy and weight loss. Baker's synovial cysts occur due to joint
complications while leg ulcers are due to the arteritis. Pernicious anaemia is an
associated autoimmune disease.

PAEDIATRICS

EXTENDED MATCHING QUESTIONS

THEME: COMMON DEVELOPMENTAL MILESTONES

1. **D** 12 months
2. **C** 9 months
3. **E** 18 months
4. **E** 18 months
5. **B** 6 months
6. **A** 3 months
7. **D** 12 months

You will need a good grasp of children's developmental milestones. At 3 months, babies can be pulled to sitting with little head lag and will hold an object placed in the hand. At 6 months, babies sit supported and transfer a cube between hands. At 9 months, they sit unsupported and may crawl on the abdomen. At 12 months, they walk with one hand held and say 2–3 words with meaning. At 18 months, they will manage a spoon, build a 3–4 cube tower, and say 10–12 words with meaning.

THEME: ABDOMINAL PAIN IN CHILDREN

8. **G** Henoch-Schönlein purpura
9. **D** Intussusception
10. **H** Appendicitis
11. **J** Testicular torsion
12. **L** Mesenteric adenitis

The purpura in HSP are classically found on extensor surfaces of the lower limbs. Treatment is supportive. The classical presentation of intussusception is rare, and it may present initially like gastroenteritis. If the appendix is retrocaecal or pelvic appendicitis may present as diarrhoea or dysuria. Urine should always be tested in children with abdominal pain. All boys with abdominal pain must have their testes examined. The danger of small bowel strangulation with inguinal hernias is high and these cases should always be referred urgently. Diabetic Ketoacidosis may cause abdominal pain which resolves on treatment with fluids and insulin.

MULTIPLE BEST ANSWER QUESTIONS

1.   Sudden Infant Death Syndrome   **Answers: C E F**
Important risk factors for Sudden Infant Death Syndrome include male sex, prone
sleeping position, the winter months and respiratory symptoms. Maternal factors
include high parity, young maternal age and smoking.

2.   Breast-feeding   **Answers: A B C**
Breast-feeding protects against respiratory disease and gastrointestinal infections. It
reduces the risk of insulin dependent diabetes and maternal breast cancer.
Childhood obesity is less likely to be found in breast-fed infants.

3.   Down's syndrome   **Answers: A C D**
40% of trisomy 21 foetuses will die between 10–14 weeks. Nuchal scanning
measures the subcutaneous oedema in the neck of the foetus using ultrasound
techniques. It is able to detect Down's syndrome *in utero* with a detection rate of
over 75%, whereas the triple test detects about 60% of cases. Ultrasound markers
with careful follow-up can detect almost 70% of cases.

4.   Breast-fed babies   **Answers: A C E**
Breast-fed babies are less likely to have gastroenteritis but no known association
with coeliac disease. Urinary tract infections are usually associated with vesico-
ureteric reflux. There is a decreased incidence of non-accidental injury, cot death
and eczema with breast-fed babies who are also less likely to be obese.

5.   Down's syndrome   **Answers: A C D**
Features in 75% of Down's include upslanting palpebral fissures, flat facies, flat
occiput and loose skin on neck. Features in 50% of Down's include broad hands,
short fingers, incurved 5th finger (clinodactyly), single palmar crease, malformed
auricles, Brushfield's spots, protruding tongue, hypotonia and broad space between
1st and 2nd toes. The IQ is usually between 20–70; average of 50.

6.   Congenital dislocation of the hip   **Answers: C D E**
Congenital dislocation of the hips is four time more common in girls, than in boys.
In doing Ortolani's test it is essential to abduct to 90°, less than 70° abduction is
abnormal. It is sometimes picked up because of delayed walking and treatment at
this stage normally requires open reduction. The best time to pick up dislocation is
as soon after birth as possible, as treatment with use of a frog plaster is always
effective.

7.   Down's syndrome   **Answers: B D**
People with Down's syndrome are prone to hypothyroidism. Clinical recognition is
difficult because people with Down's syndrome are shorter than average, slower,
less active and less alert and occasionally have a hoarse voice. Post-mortem studies
of people with Down's syndrome have confirmed that a high proportion have
pathological changes indistinguishable from Alzheimer's disease.

8.   Nocturnal enuresis   **Answers: A C**

90% of children with nocturnal enuresis are dry during the day. First born children appear to be more prone to nocturnal enuresis than later children. By the age of 10 years, 7% of children still wet their beds at least once a week. Urodynamic studies do not often help diagnose the cause of nocturnal enuresis. It is not known how the tricyclic antidepressants (e.g. imipramine) achieve temporary dryness, but it does not seem to be related to their anticholinergic or antidepressant effect or their local anaesthetic effect on the bladder.

9.   Baby of eight months   **Answers: A C**

Rolling over is acquired by most babies at five months of age. The ability to pick up a bead between finger and thumb is usually only evident at about one year. Babies sit unsupported at eight months. Babies usually feed themselves with a spoon after one year. Most babies say their first words clearly around 12–14 months, but five words will often not be clearly spoken until 14–16 months.

SINGLE BEST ANSWER QUESTIONS

1.   Congenital dislocation of the hip   **Answer: C**

The incidence of congenital dislocation of the hip is 2–3 per 1000 births. Screening may not be worthwhile – the rate of surgical intervention has not decreased with screening. Splinting can be associated with avascular necrosis of the femoral head.

2.   Congenital dislocation of the hip   **Answer: A**

Congenital dislocation of hips is seen in about 0.25% of newborns with a female to male predominance of 8:1. Most are unilateral and usually are on the left. 90% of dislocatable hips will stabilise in first two months of life. However, the ones which will stabilize cannot be predicted so all patients are treated with a flexion-abduction-external rotation device. Ultrasound of the hips is very useful in making the diagnosis in the newborn. Femoral head ossification centres appear at 3–6 months so radiographs are not useful in the newborn. The most significant risk factor for hip dysplasia is a positive family history. Other risk factors for hip dysplasia include breech presentation, foot deformities, oligohydramnios, primiparity and female sex.

3.   Puberty   **Answer: A**

Menarche is a late event in puberty. On average there is only 2 inches (5cm) of growth potential remaining after menarche. The pubertal growth spurt in normal girls always occurs earlier. Delayed pubertal development is most commonly due to physiological delay in development, hallmarked by short stature, delayed adrenarche, delayed gonadarche and a retarded bone age. The commonest cause of central precocious puberty in girls is 'idiopathic'. In boys the commonest cause is a CNS lesion.

4.   Infantile colic   Answer: E

A recent review of the trial data in clinical evidence suggest that behavioural modification involving less stimulation by the parents was the only effective treatment. Dicyclomine may be effective but has adverse effects. There is no evidence of dietary modification making a difference.

PHARMACO-THERAPEUTICS

EXTENDED MATCHING QUESTIONS

THEME: SIMILAR SOUNDING DRUGS

1. **E** Loratidine
2. **C** Loperamide
3. **A** Lansoprazole
4. **D** Loprazolan
5. **F** Lorezepam
6. **E** Loratidine
7. **A** Lansoprazole
8. **B** Lofepramine

Some questions about drugs can be answered easily. Loratidine is an antihistamine and can be used in the symptomatic treatment of urticaria. Loperamide is used as an adjunct to rehydration in acute diarrhoea and can cause abdominal cramps. Lansoprazole is a proton pump inhibitor and can be used in the treatment of duodenal ulcers. Loprazolan is a hypnotic. Lorezepam is an anxiolytic and can be used in the treatment of status epilepticus. Lofepramine is an antidepressant.

THEME: SIDE-EFFECTS OF DYSPEPSIA TREATMENT

9. **E** Misoprostol
10. **E** Misoprostol
11. **C** Magnesium salts
12. **F** Omeprazole
13. **A** Aluminium salts
14. **D** Metoclopramide
15. **D** Metoclopramide
16. **B** H_2-receptor antagonists

The side-effects of common treatments ought to be familiar. Misoprostol can cause intermenstrual bleeding and can be associated with postmenopausal bleeding. Aluminium salts frequently causes constipation, while magnesium salts are frequently associated with diarrhoea. Omeprazole can cause severe skin reactions and photosensitivity. Metoclopramide is associated with dystonic reactions and can cause galactorrhoea. H_2-receptor antagonists can cause confusion, which is reversible on stopping the medication.

THEME: ANTI-INFECTIVE DRUG SIDE-EFFECTS

17. **H** Acyclovir
18. **C** Zanamavir
19. **D** Doxycycline
20. **G** Rifampicin
21. **A** Ciprofloxacin
22. **F** Metronidazole

Long-term treatment with acyclovir in the prophylaxis of recurrent herpes simplex infections requires regular monitoring of renal function. Relenza should not be used in severe asthmatics and patients with mild asthma should be advised to keep a bronchodilator to hand. Patients on doxycycline should be warned about the risk of sunburn, particularly when used for malarial prophylaxis. Patients being treated for TB or meningococcal prophylaxis should be warned about staining of contact lenses. The elderly and those on steroids are particularly prone to tendon damage. The CSM advise stopping quinolones at the first signs of tendon inflammation. They are contraindicated in pregnant women and children. Metronidazole may cause severe nausea and vomiting if taken with alcohol. Ciprofloxacin may potentiate the effects of alcohol.

MULTIPLE BEST ANSWER QUESTIONS

1. Renal failure   Answers: B E
Tetracyclines, apart from doxycycline, should be avoided in renal failure as they are antianabolic, causing salt and water loss, raise the blood urea and can lead to permanent loss of nephrons in the kidney. Nitrofurantoin is prone to give toxic levels and peripheral neuropathy in renal failure. It is also likely to be ineffective for urinary infections. Although aluminium hydroxide is used for phosphate lowering, there are concerns about aluminium retention with prolonged usage.

2. Benzodiazepine anxiolytics   Answers: B D
There is little difference in the pharmacodynamics of the many available benzodiazepines. They do however differ in their duration of action. Temazepam and oxazepam are short-acting, whereas diazepam and its active metabolites persist in the body for a long time with a half-time of up to three days in the elderly. The increase in body sway predisposes to falls, especially in the elderly.

3. Cannabis   Answers: A D
Cannabis is usually smoked but can be ingested or injected intravenously. The clinical features of cannabis intake include euphoria with drowsiness, distorted and heightened images, altered tactile sensations, tachycardia, hypertension and ataxia with visual and auditory hallucinations. Injections may produce nausea and vomiting within minutes and, after about an hour, profuse watery diarrhoea.

4. Aspirin
Answers: A C

Aspirin in large doses is hypoprothrombinaemic. In smaller doses, it increases the bleeding tendency by its antiplatelet and gastric irritant effects. Also, in large doses, aspirin is uricosuric, but in therapeutic doses of 1–2 g/day or less, it reduces urate excretion.

5. Renal failure
Answers: A C E

Aspirin causes sodium and water retention, deterioration in renal function and increased risk of gastro-intestinal bleeding. Avoid glibenclamide in severe renal impairment, because of increased risk of hypoglycaemia. Muscle toxicities may occur with all statins, particularly in patients with renal impairment.

6. Cannabis abuse
Answers: C D

Chronic cannabis abuse produces reversible intellectual impairment. Initial reports of cerebral atrophy have not been confirmed. Cannabis smoke may be carcinogenic.

7. Side-effects of benzodiazepines
Answers: A B C

Benzodiazepines are anxiolytic, sedative, anticonvulsants and act as a muscle relaxant. Benzodiazepines are well tolerated and side-effects tend to be a result of overdosage which leads to drowsiness and confused thinking especially in the elderly. They potentiate the effects of central nervous system depressants such as alcohol.

8. Warfarin
Answers: A D E

The main interactions with warfarin are due either to hepatic enzyme inhibition (e.g. cimetidine, cotrimoxazole) or to enzyme induction (e.g. rifampicin, phenytoin). Non-steroidal anti-inflammatory drugs may predispose to gastric erosion and ulceration, with consequent risk of GI bleeding.

9. Breast-feeding women
Answers: D E

Sulphonamides are unsuitable because they may cause kernicterus. Aspirin is not to be used because it may cause Reye's syndrome and lithium should be avoided because it may result in cardiovascular collapse.

10. Combined oral contraceptive pill
Answers: A B E

The effectiveness of the combined pill can be reduced by antibiotics, some tranquillisers and anticonvulsants, and griseofulvin. Rifamycin accelerates metabolism of the pill and reduces its effect, as does carbamazepine and griseofulvin. The pill antagonises the anticoagulant effect of warfarin and antagonises hypotensive effect of lisinopril.

11. Drugs in pregnancy
Answers: A D E

With piperazine there is no clinical evidence of harm but packs sold to the public carry a warning to avoid the drug in pregnancy except on medical advice. Avoid simvastatin since congenital anomalies have been reported (the decreased synthesis of cholesterol possibly affects fetal development). Avoid enalapril since it may adversely affect fetal and neonatal blood pressure control and renal function. Also, there are possible skull defects and oligohydramnios. There is no evidence of teratogenicity with chlorpheniramine and paracetamol. However, it is wise to err on the side of caution and give only essential medication to pregnant women.

12. Non-steroidal anti-inflammatory drugs   Answers: D E
Hyperkalaemia is linked with non-steroidal anti-inflammatory drugs (NSAIDs). Haemolytic anaemia, rather than polycythaemia, is linked with usage of NSAIDs.

SINGLE BEST ANSWER QUESTIONS

1. Drugs contraindicated in breast-feeding   Answer: B
Most drugs enter breast milk by passive lipid diffusion. As the plasma drug concentration is relatively low compared to total body concentration, the load to the baby is small. It is wise to be cautious, but only drugs known to be toxic to the child should be avoided completely. Senna can cause increased gastric mobility and diarrhoea.

2. Zanamivir (Relenza)   Answer: B
Zanamivir (Relenza) probably affects neuraminidase activity and so inhibits replication of Influenza virus (types A and B). It has to be taken as a nasal spray or dry powder inhalation, and its effect is greatest in those patients seen within 30 hours. It does enable a quicker return to work but may possibly exacerbate asthma.

3. St. John's wort   Answer: A
St John's wort is used commonly in the UK, and has been shown to be effective in treating depression. It can induce liver enzymes and can interact with digoxin, warfarin and the pill.

4. Digoxin therapy   Answer: D
Old people are at risk of toxicity especially with hypokalaemia or hypercalcaemia. Almost any arrhythmia (usually SVT with AV block) will occur. Other symptoms include decreased cognition, yellow-green visual halos, nausea and vomiting. Prolonged PR interval is noted with first-degree heart block.

5. Warfarin   Answer: D
All broad spectrum antibiotics including ampicillin can increase the prothrombin time. In drug interactions with warfarin, consider these effects.

- Displacement of warfarin from the protein binding site by for example sulphonamides, NSAIDs and sulphonylureas. A new steady state is then established. Consequently, the danger is at the start or end of therapy.
- Enzyme inhibition or competition (e.g. cimetidine)
- Enzyme induction (e.g. rifampicin, griseofulvin and carbamazepine)

6.   Glibenclamide   **Answer: A**

Glibenclamide has a relatively long biological half-life although it is shorter than chlorpropamide. Unfortunately, it also has biologically active metabolites with a long half-life which are excreted by the kidney. This therefore precludes the use of glibenclamide in patients with renal impairment. It should be used with caution in the elderly. Despite strong protein binding, all sulphonylureas cross the placenta, producing foetal hyperinsulinaemia and predisposing to macrosomia and neonatal hypoglycaemia.

PSYCHIATRY/ NEUROLOGY

EXTENDED MATCHING QUESTIONS

THEME: SECTIONS OF THE MENTAL HEALTH ACT

1. **E** Section 7
2. **B** Section 3
3. **C** Section 4
4. **D** Section 5
5. **A** Section 2

Some knowledge of the Mental Health Act is desirable. Section 2 is used for assessment, section 3 for treatment. Section 4 and 5 are both emergency detention orders; section 4 is used to admit someone to hospital and section 5 is used to keep someone in hospital. Section 7 is concerned with guardianship.

THEME: HEADACHES

6. **B** Migraine
7. **D** Tension headaches
8. **D** Tension headaches
9. **B** Migraine
10. **A** Cluster headaches

Patients with tension headaches often describe the pain as a weight on the top of the head or as a band. Headache that is pain referred from the neck may be associated with certain movements, postures or positions. With migraine the patient will commonly show pallor and often experiences flushing. Cluster headaches are frequently accompanied by the complaint of a watery eye.

THEME: DISC LESIONS

11. **B** At L5–S1 level
12. **C** Central disc prolapse
13. **A** At L2–L3 level

Patients with disc lesions at the L2–L3 level will usually demonstrate a positive femoral stretch test. At the L5–S1 level there will be loss of the ankle reflex. With a central disc prolapse there will usually be loss of bladder function.

THEME: QUESTIONNAIRES

14. A CAGE
15. E SCOFF
16. B MAST
17. A CAGE

MAST and CAGE are commonly used questionnaires in detecting alcohol problems. MAST asks 10 questions and has a maximum score of **32.** The questions include questions about alcohol-related driving and hospital admissions. CAGE is a very short questionnaire with only four questions, but it is significant if any two questions are positive. SCOFF is used in eating disorders. EAT is not a questionnaire; it is an Employment Appeal Tribunal.

THEME: HEADACHE

18. B Tension headache
19. I Coital cephalgia
20. A Cluster headache
21. G Migraine without aura
22. C Temporal arteritis
23. D Migraine with aura

One of the key points in the history of tension headache is that it occurs at times of stress and gets better on relaxation, e.g. on holiday. Coital cephalgia is rare; onset is during intercourse. The clinical pictures may be similar to that of subarachnoid haemorrhage and CSF examination may be necessary to differentiate the two. Cluster headache is seen in a sex ratio of 7:1, male:female and produces bouts of pain from 20–60 minutes long, occurring at the same time each day. There may be associated facial flushing, nasal secretion or even an ipsilateral Horner's syndrome. Alcohol may provoke attacks. Giant cell arteritis typically affects the elderly who may present with symptoms of polymyalgia rheumatica. Early diagnosis and treatment with high dose steroids is crucial in preserving sight.

THEME: PSYCHIATRIC COMPLAINTS

24. I Dementia
25. D Conversion disorder
26. J Anxiety disorder
27. C Borderline personality disorder
28. G Bipolar disorder
29. H Schizophrenia

Dementia typically causes loss of short-term memory first, and socially skilled patients may confabulate to get around this. Mood disorders may appear and family relationships are often strained by inability to carry out simple tasks. Conversion disorder often represents a patient's idea of what the disease looks like, hence symptoms and signs seldom match. There is usually some gain for the patient and they may seem remarkably unfazed by events, 'la belle indifférence'. Anxiety disorders often start after a stressful life event, and attacks consist of psychological symptoms of fearful anticipation and worry, and physical symptoms. The symptoms of borderline personality disorder are similar to those for antisocial personality disorder. The symptoms of the manic phase in bipolar disorder are similar in some respects to hyperthyroidism and this should be excluded.

THEME: MIGRAINE

30. **B** Aspirin
31. **F** Avoidance of trigger factors
32. **C** PR diclofenac
33. **E** Sumatriptan
34. **I** Ergotamine
35. **H** Emergency medical referral

A stepwise approach to migraine treatment starts with over the counter remedies such as aspirin as step 1. Step 2 involves parenteral routes. If migraines are not controlled on this step the next treatment is sumatriptan. If sumatriptan does not control symptoms the diagnosis should be reviewed. Ergotamine is a step 4 treatment. At any time alternative diagnoses should be considered, particularly subarachnoid haemorrhage or meningitis. Opiates and opioids should never be used due to potential for addiction and poor efficacy.

THEME: HEADACHES

36. **G** Temporal arteritis
37. **F** Migraine
38. **A** Alcoholism
39. **E** Depression
40. **C** Carbon monoxide poisoning

The answer requires the most likely diagnosis. Each of the histories could possibly have more than one answer, but the question is specific. Although the middle-aged GP may have a brain tumour, it is far more likely that he is a drinker. The young girl moving in with her boyfriend is possibly going to get migraine from the oral contraceptive pill, while the patient who has just moved house may have a faulty central heating boiler.

THEME: MRC SCALE FOR MUSCLE POWER

41. E 3
42. C 1
43. H 5

In the MRC scale for muscle power, 5 = normal power, 3 = movement overcomes gravity plus added resistance, and 1 = no movement of joint but muscle contraction visible.

THEME: NERVE ROOT LESIONS

44. G S1/S2
45. B C5
46. C C6
47. E L3/4

You need to know about innervations of reflexes and muscles. Although these can vary somewhat the clinical scenarios will be specific.

Biceps reflex = C5
Supinator reflex = C6
Triceps reflex = C6/C7
Knee reflex = L3/L4
Ankle reflex = S1

MULTIPLE BEST ANSWER QUESTIONS

1. Essential tremor   Answers: B D
Essential tremor is most pronounced with outstretched arms (sustained posture) and is typically relieved by alcohol. A Parkinson's disease tremor is most pronounced at rest and is a cerebellar tremor with movement (intention). Anxiety may exacerbate both essential and Parkinson's disease tremor.

2. Risk factors for suicide   Answers: A D E F
Risk factors for suicide include a history of recent self harm, the severity of depressive illness, and the presence of active plans. Being male, unemployed and single are also risk factors.

3. Major depression   Answers: B C E
A working class background predisposes to major depression. The loss of a parent in childhood and the presence of several children in the house also predispose to an episode of major depression. Unemployment, rather than continuous employment, is a major factor in the aetiology of depression.

4. Compensation neurosis · Answers: B E

The incidence of compensation neurosis has an inverse relationship with the severity of the injury. It is twice as common after industrial injuries as after road traffic accidents. Little recovery is found in patients with severe symptoms even after settlement of the compensation claim. The main symptoms are headaches, dizziness, poor concentration and irritability. Malingering is not a common occurrence, and the mechanisms involved in producing these symptoms appear to be subconscious ones.

5. Agoraphobia · Answers: B C D

Agoraphobia generally commences suddenly in adult life following a recent traumatic event. There is a large preponderance of women patients, and a worsening of symptoms can occur as a result of other emotional changes such as a period of depression. Treatment is very difficult, but the condition can respond to desensitisation by systematically introducing the patient to the feared situation.

6. Grief reaction · Answers: A B D

The initial stage of a grief reaction is a period of numbness with little or no emotional reaction. This is the period of denial. Subsequent stages follow to a state of depression, and suicidal ideas are often expressed. These may reflect feelings of guilt or identification with the dead person. The reaction is self-limiting although there may be delays up to several years. The treatment of choice would be some form of psychotherapy or counselling. The grief reaction is a neurotic illness rather than psychotic.

7. Anxiety states · Answers: A E

Many physical symptoms are associated with anxiety states: dyspnoea, difficulty inhaling, overbreathing, dry mouth, difficulty swallowing, palpitations, chest pain, frequency and urgency of micturition, tinnitus, blurred vision, paraesthesia, dizziness and sweating. Difficulty concentrating and complaints of poor memory occur. Persistent and objective memory loss is not present and raises the possibility of an organic cause. Depressive illnesses may present with anxiety symptoms; low mood and early morning wakening would be indicative of this. Problems getting to sleep are more usual with anxiety disorders.

8. Obsessive-compulsive disorder · Answers: A E

Obsessive-compulsive disorders are characterised by obsessional thinking and compulsive behaviour. Obsessional thoughts are words, ideas or beliefs that intrude into the patient's mind. They are recognised as the patient's own thoughts. They are usually unpleasant, are resisted and are associated with anxiety. Obsessional thoughts lead to obsessional actions which may reduce anxiety. Obsessional ruminations are endless internal debates, sometimes about insignificant details. Anxiety and depression are commonly associated. Men and women are equally affected. Two-thirds improve by the end of a year, cases of more than one year run a fluctuating course.

9.   Schizophrenia   Answers: A D E

In the absence of coarse brain disease the presence of Schneider's first rank symptoms point to a diagnosis of schizophrenia. They are:

1.   Specific types of auditory hallucination (audible thoughts, voices talking about the patient in the third person, voices commenting on actions (running commentary))
2.   Passivity phenomena (breakdown of ego-boundaries), thought insertion, withdrawal and broadcast, forced acts and feelings (somatic passivity)
3.   Delusions (primary delusions or delusional perceptions)

10.   Acute confusional state   Answers: C D E

Almost every disease, bodily insult and drug has been credited with precipitating acute confusion. Commonly implicated factors are trauma, surgery, heart failure, infection, anoxia and sedative drugs. Confusion is not, however, a characteristic feature of myxoedema. Dementia is a very common predisposing condition and tricyclics may precipitate a confusional state. Phenothiazines such as thioridazine may be used therapeutically but dealing with the precipitating factor is most important.

11.   Hypomania   Answers: A C E

Flight of ideas, where there is an excessively fluent flow of thoughts and ideas, but with some thread of connection between them, is characteristic of hypomania. Thought insertion is a first rank symptom of schizophrenia. Overactivity and a sense of grandiosity can lead to sexually promiscuous behaviour. Delusions of bodily illness are a feature of depression, not mania. The manic patient is so active he/she tends to have very little sleep and can become ill through exhaustion.

12.   Alcohol withdrawal   Answers: A B D

Delirium tremens on withdrawal from alcohol includes a coarse, persistent tremor of the hands. Often, the patient experiences visual hallucinations such as seeing animals crawling on the floor or the bedclothes. There is free perspiration, oliguria and dehydration. Passivity feelings are features of schizophrenia. Confabulation is part of Korsakoff's syndrome resulting from chronic alcohol abuse and is not a feature of acute withdrawal.

13.   Hysteria   Answers: B C

A hysterical symptom is one that suggests physical illness but occurs in the absence of physical disease and is not produced deliberately. Hysterical symptoms occur in association with several psychiatric disorders: depression, anxiety and organic mental disorder. 'La belle indifference' is a characteristic, but is not always present. Hysterical symptoms developing for the first time in middle or old age should raise a high suspicion of organic disease. There are usually obvious discrepancies between signs and symptoms of hysteria and those of organic disease, although this depends on the patient's medical knowledge.

14. Suicide
Answers: A D F G

Tactful enquiry about suicidal intent may decrease the risk of suicide. The following factors are associated with an increased risk of suicide: male sex, old age, alcohol abuse, drug dependence, epilepsy, chronic physical illness (especially chronic painful conditions), bereavement, social isolation, psychiatric disorder (apart from obsessional illness), family history of suicide or depression, previous suicide attempts and unemployment.

15. Schizophrenia
Answers: B D

Schizophrenia with an early onset usually results in a more chronic deterioration in personality. Affective change, like depression, appears to indicate some preservation of personality and a better prognosis. Individual symptoms such as visual hallucinations do not appear to influence prognosis. Echolalia usually indicates an organic brain problem.

16. Multiple sclerosis
Answers: B D

Multiple sclerosis (MS) has a higher prevalence in temperate than in tropical countries. Japanese have an exceptionally low incidence. MS may present with diplopia but it is due to involvement of cranial nerves III, IV or VI, not the optic nerve. MS quite frequently causes sensory disturbance of the limbs.

17. Bell's palsy
Answers: B D E

Dry eye caused by denervation of the lacrimal gland is very uncommon, whereas a watering eye is common. The salivary glands are not affected in Bell's palsy. Postauricular pain is common and may actually precede paralysis.

18. In the leg
Answers: A B E

In the arm, spasticity in a patient with hemiplegia is most pronounced in the flexor muscles and weakness in the extensor muscles. The converse is true in the leg. The peroneal nerve supplies skin over the lateral aspect of the lower leg. The saphenous branch of the femoral nerve supplies skin over the medial aspect of the lower leg. A femoral nerve palsy causes weakness of knee extensions. A sciatic nerve palsy causes weakness of hip extension, knee flexion and foot dorsiflexion, plantar flexion, inversion and eversion.

19. Multiple sclerosis
Answers: B E

The diagnosis of multiple sclerosis (MS) is predominantly a clinical one requiring discrete lesions in time and space. Investigations only aid in confirming your suspicion. Magnetic resonance imaging has become the investigation of choice. Visual evoked potentials can be measured and are abnormal even in the absence of previous optic neuritis. Both hemianopia and dysphasia are extremely rare manifestations of MS. Epilepsy is more common, occurring in approximately 5% as a late complication. Red and green colour impairment or dimming of vision are common sequelae of optic neuritis. Bad prognostic signs are being male, onset after 40 years, predominant motor signs, poor recovery between each relapse and a short interval between each episode.

20.   Stroke   **Answers: A B**

Stroke is more common in people in lower socio-economic groups, probably because they smoke more and are more likely to suffer from hypertension. About 50% of patients with intracerebral or subarachnoid haemorrhage die within 30 days of their stroke, while in cerebral infarction the mortality is only 10%. Hypertension is the most important risk factor for stroke.

SINGLE BEST ANSWER QUESTIONS

1.   Alzheimer's disease   **Answer: F**

Alzheimer's disease is the most common cause of dementia. Amnesia and spatial dysfunction are typical early clinical features and social graces are usually maintained until late in the disease. The underlying pathology predominantly affects the temporal and parietal cortices. Extrapyramidal rigidity, long tract signs and myoclonus are all late clinical manifestations. The EEG is typically abnormal.

2.   Differential diagnosis of dementia   **Answer: D**

The incidence of multi-infarct dementia varies greatly in different series. This is undoubtedly due to the lack of a good differentiation test between this and Alzheimer's disease. If a gait disturbance or urinary incontinence appears early in the course of a dementing illness, normal pressure hydrocephalus should be considered. The presence of any symptoms or signs which may arise from subcortical structures should alert the clinician to diagnoses other than the pure cortical dementias (e.g. Wilson's disease, Huntington's disease or Parkinson's disease may need to be considered).

The rapid progression of a dementing process with associated long tract signs, myoclonic jerks and severe rigidity point to the possibility of Creutzfeldt-Jakob disease. An EEG is abnormal in approximately 90% of cases of Creutzfeldt-Jakob disease, showing characteristic changes.

3.   Alcohol   **Answer: B**

The relationship between alcohol and risk of death is complicated; the lowest risk appears to be in those who consume 7–21 units per week. A combination of a raised MCV and a raised gamma GT will pick up 90% of problem drinkers. A similar proportion will answer yes to two of the five CAGE questions.

4.   Risk of suicide   **Answer: E**

The most obvious warning sign of suicide is a direct statement of intent by the patient. There is no truth in the theory that people who talk about killing themselves actually do not do it. The presence of a feeling of hopelessness is a predictor of both immediate and subsequent suicide. Of the social factors, positive family history of suicide, prolonged physical illness and living alone indicate a higher risk. Paranoid delusions can occur in depressive illness, but do not have any special significance in assessing suicide risk.

171

5.   Chronic fatigue syndrome   Answer: B
Few risk factors have been identified for chronic fatigue syndrome apart from previous psychiatric illness. More than 75% of affected patients have a concurrent psychiatric illness, depression being present in more than half. No relationship has been demonstrated between clinical status and any laboratory findings. The treatment of choice appears to be a structured return to physical activity and cognitive behavioural therapy, with treatment of any associated depression.

6.   Tricyclic antidepressants   Answer: C
Tricyclic antidepressants take at least ten days to have their effect. They have no interaction with food unlike the monoamineoxidase inhibitors. The tricyclic antidepressants do not induce sensitivity to sunlight unlike the phenothiazines. The tricyclic antidepressants have no direct effect on weight, except that as the depression resolves, the appetite should improve. Initial side-effects include dry mouth, but this usually clears up after a few days. Patients should be given this information so that they are encouraged to persist with treatment.

7.   Tricyclic antidepressants   Answer: D
The tricyclic antidepressants have a number of important side-effects. They can produce dry mouth, blurred vision, urinary retention, constipation, postural hypotension, tachycardia and increased sweating. They can also cause fine tremor, unco-ordination, headaches, epileptic fits and peripheral neuropathy. Tricyclics are contraindicated in glaucoma. Tricyclic antidepressants may be used in patients with ischaemic heart disease, with caution. They are safe in patients anticoagulated with warfarin.

8.   Post-herpetic neuralgia   Answer: D
Gabapentin and amitryptyline are both effective for post herpetic neuralgia. Topical capsaicin is effective but may cause skin irritation. Epidural morphine is effective but not appropriate for the majority of patients.

9.   Motor neurone disease   Answer: A
As the name motor neurone disease implies, degeneration occurs in the motor neurones. One group of motor neurones has its origin in the motor and pre-motor cortex, terminating in the brain stem or spinal cord. The second group has its origin in the brain stem or spinal cord, terminating in the muscle fibres.

10.   Multiple sclerosis   Answer: E
Of the treatments mentioned, the only treatment proved to reduce the severity of relapse in multiple sclerosis is dietary supplementation with linoleic acid. Trials have shown both azathioprine and hyperbaric oxygen to be ineffective and potentially dangerous. Corticosteroids and ACTH bring forward remission following relapse but do not modify the overall course of the disease.

11. Migraine **Answer: A**

Migraine without aura occurs in 75% of patients. Daily headaches are never migrainous. Although migrainous headaches are usually unilateral, they can occasionally be bilateral. Migrainous attacks are probably caused by the release of vasogenic amines from blood vessel walls accompanied by pulsatile distension.

12. Backache **Answer: D**

Symptoms of nerve root irritation, such as unilateral leg pain worse than back pain and pain radiating to the buttocks do not need specialist referral. Perineal anaesthesia, sphincter disturbance or gait disturbance are neurosurgical emergencies and require immediate referral. Presentation under 20 or over 55 may indicate malignancy and prompt referral (less than four weeks) should be considered. (RCGP guidelines.)

REPRODUCTIVE/ RENAL

EXTENDED MATCHING QUESTIONS

THEME: COMMON CANCERS

1. **A** Breast cancer
2. **A** Breast cancer
3. **C** Endometrial cancer
4. **D** Ovarian cancer
5. **B** Cervical cancer
6. **B** Cervical cancer

Look carefully at clinical scenario questions for the hints that will give you the 'correct' answer. The most common malignant tumour that affects women only is breast cancer, which is also associated with an early menarche, rapid establishment of regular menstruation, obesity and high alcohol intake. Endometrial cancer is linked with unopposed oestrogen use and progestagen oral contraception may be protective. Ovarian cancer is more common in nulliparous and subfertile women, and sometimes has a familial tendency. Cervical cancer is linked with early teenage sexual intercourse, increased parity, smoking and has been linked to oral contraceptive use of more than 10 years.

THEME: MENSTRUAL DISTURBANCES

7. **C** Cervical erosion
8. **F** Climacteric
9. **A** Fibroids
10. **E** Endometriosis
11. **H** Polycystic ovary disease
12. **D** Normal menstrual cycle

Cervical erosions occur at times of high oestrogen levels, such as pregnancy, puberty and the pill. Non-offensive clear discharge and occasional post-coital spotting may occur. Cryocautery may be used if the discharge is troublesome. The climacteric is characterised by irregular cycles, hot flushes, intermittently heavy bleeds and mood changes. The mean age of onset in the UK is 51 (range 40–57). Fibroids are benign smooth muscle tumours, commoner in Africans and enlarge slowly in pregnancy and on the pill. Symptoms are due to a mass effect (frequency and distension) and an increase in endometrial surface area (menorrhagia).

Endometriosis is typically seen in 30–45 year old women with dysmenorrhoea, menorrhagia, dyspareunia and infertility. PCOS classically causes infertility, obesity, hirsutism and menstrual disturbances. It can be diagnosed clinically, by ultrasound or with a raised LH/FSH ratio. The 'normal' intermenstrual interval of 28 days is only seen in 12% of women not on the pill. Asking patients to keep a diary over 3–4 cycles will often confirm regular cycles.

THEME: CONTRACEPTION

13. **B** Minipill
14. **G** Implanon
15. **D** IUD Insertion
16. **I** Depo-Provera
17. **E** Diaphragm
18. **H** Mirena IUS

The combined pill is contraindicated in women over 35 who smoke and have high blood pressure. The minipill is the best choice in this situation as its effectiveness in terms of pregnancies in users per year is very good in older women. This will give her time to think about future options e.g. sterilization. A good choice here in travellers would be implanon. Starting the pill now would not allow follow up, and she is concerned about DVT. Depo-Provera only lasts 12 weeks. Implanon provides 3 years protection and is easily reversible. It does however require skilled insertion and removal. For emergency contraception speed is of the essence. After 72 hours the only option is IUD insertion which may be done up to 5 days after intercourse. Focal migraine and ergotamine both preclude the use of oestrogenic contraceptives due to a risk of stroke. The minipill is not particularly effective in younger users and must be taken at the same time each day. Depo-Provera is highly effective and easy to use. The diaphragm in combination with spermicide may be an effective choice for women approaching the menopause who still require contraception. Mirena offers excellent contraception and the majority are amennorhoeic within 6 months. It works for 5 years.

MULTIPLE BEST ANSWER QUESTIONS

1. Postnatal depression   Answers: B D
Postnatal depression affects over 10% of all deliveries but is often undetected. It is more common when there is a past psychiatric history. About 1/3 cases become chronic. Antidepressants are used in treatment with no evidence for benefit from hormonal therapy.

2. Postnatal depression   Answers: A B
Postnatal depression occurs in up to 25% of women after giving birth and is more common in women with a history of psychiatric illness. Surprisingly, women who have had obstetric complications do not seem to suffer more from postnatal depression. Suicide attempts by women shortly after birth are very rare.

Antidepressant drugs are secreted only in small amounts into breast milk so treatment by them using moderate dosages is safe.

3.   Breast-feeding   Answers: B C D
Human milk is low in protein compared with cows' milk, but cows' milk and human milk have similar fat contents. Hindmilk is more nutritious than foremilk, containing twice as much fat on average. Vitamin K levels in breast milk are low, which perhaps explains why haemorrhagic disease of the newborn is most common in breast-fed babies. An exclusively breast-fed infant will start becoming short of iron at about 6 months.

4.   Hormone Replacement Therapy   Answers: A C
HRT invariably reduces hot flushes and has been shown to reduce risk of osteoporosis. Weight gain is a possibility, but more often it is a question of weight redistribution. Improvement in libido can happen, but not in the majority. The risk of breast cancer is greater with family history or previous lumps.

5.   Chlamydia infections   Answers: C D
Chlamydia infections are found in about 5% of women attending General Practitioners; it is the commonest curable STD in the developed world. 75% of cases seem to be asymptomatic but long-term effects are infertility and ectopic pregnancy. Screening can be difficult but it appears to be possible using urine samples.

6.   Carcinoma of the cervix   Answers: A B
There has been a large increase in the number of women having cervical smears and a steady fall in both incidence and mortality from cervical cancer. HPV is sexually transmitted and a strong link with cervical cancer exists, in that almost all cases of cervical cancer have HPV infection. However, most women with HPV infection will not develop cancer of the cervix.

7.   Contraception   Answers: A B C D
The pill has many positive advantages in addition to its contraceptive effect. It suppresses both benign breast disease and ovarian cysts. It also decreases the rate of pelvic inflammatory disease and ovarian cancer. However, use of the pill does increase the risk of pulmonary embolism, arterial disease and possibly increases the risk of breast cancer.

8.   Hormone replacement therapy   Answers: C D E
Most of the work on hormone replacement therapy comes from observational studies. There is a problem with bias because of the population taking HRT. Hormone replacement therapy appears to control most menopausal symptoms but not peri-menopausal depression. HRT prevents osteoporosis and this effect is enhanced by calcium supplements. Women taking HRT live longer but this may be due to the bias in women that take the HRT. On the negative side, however, there appears to be a slightly increased incidence of DVTs in women taking HRT.

9. Hormonal post-coital contraception
Answers: B E

A short course of high dose progestogen is more reliable as a post-coital contraception than a mixture of oestrogen and progestogen. The first dose is taken as soon as possible after unprotected intercourse, the second dose 12 hours later. It can be up to 72 hours but has greater efficacy if taken soon after unprotected intercourse. If there is any vomiting, the dose should be repeated immediately. One should exclude pregnancy if periods are delayed.

10. Antenatal women
Answers: A C E

Women are best advised to take folic acid from pre-conception for the first trimester – 5 mg a day if the previous baby had neural tube defects and 0.4 mg for others. Increased vitamins from diet are usually sufficient and the addition of multivitamin supplements has little effect. Moreover, vitamin A in high doses can be teratogenic. Giving all pregnant women iron supplements is not advised unless the mother has true iron deficiency. Soft ripened cheeses such as brie and camembert should not be eaten during pregnancy; hard cheeses can be eaten. Pates may be contaminated with listeria.

11. Causes of menorrhagia
Answers: B C D

Causes also include polyps, endometrial cancer, dysfunctional uterine bleeding, endometriosis and blood dyscrasias. Psychological causes can be implicated since the perception of blood loss is very subjective. Myxodema rather than thyrotoxicosis is associated with menorrhagia. Fibroids can be associated with menorrhagia presumably due to the increased surface area of the endometrium. The IUCD causes direct effects that result in menorrhagia. Anorexia and thyrotoxicosis usually cause amenorrhoea.

12. Pre-eclampsia
Answers: A C D

Pre-disposition to pre-eclampsia occurs in diabetics, primigravida and twin pregnancies (possibly due to the large placenta). Hydatidiform moles are associated with an increased incidence of pre-eclampsia.

13. Contraception counselling
Answers: B C

Gillick ruling allowed doctors legally to provide contraception to girls under 16, without parental consent. It is not always essential to take a full sexual history, but important facts need to be established and realisation of under age sex needs to be kept in mind. It is not recommended to use IUCD or Mirena.

14. Puerperal psychosis
Answers: B E F

Puerperal psychosis usually begins within the first two weeks. There are three main types of clinical picture: acute organic, affective (depressive or manic) and schizophrenic. The most common presentation is depressive. The onset is usually acute and the prognosis good. The risk of recurrence in subsequent pregnancies is between 1:3 and 1:7.

15. Perimenopausal contraception
Answers: B D

FSH levels are reliable in progesterone only pill users, but not in combined pill users. IUCD is a possibility, including Mirena.

16. Puerperal psychosis
Answers: B C D

The majority of puerperal psychoses begin within the first two weeks after childbirth, and rarely in the first two days. The illness usually starts with a period of delirium. The outlook is favourable. Auditory hallucinations are frequently experienced, but obsessional ruminations are not part of the clinical picture.

17. Torsion of the testis
Answers: A B D

Torsion of the testis is most common in the 12–22 age group; generally after a physical injury, usually from sport. It usually presents with abdominal pain and vomiting and always requires urgent referral, as delay can cause non-viable testis. At operation, if the testis is non-viable it should always be removed, as antibodies will cause infertility. An average General Practitioner is more than likely to see at least one case in their lifetime.

18. Benign prostatic hypertrophy
Answers: A C

The prevalence of BPH is increasing as the population is ageing and more patients are reporting symptoms. Nocturia is a very poor diagnostic feature, as this can be caused by multiple reasons including insomnia, or large fluid intake. Beta-blockers remain drugs of choice, despite the fact that they do not reduce the size of the prostate gland. The number of TURPs have more than halved in the last ten years. PSA test should only be offered to patients after careful counselling in selected groups.

19. Prostatic cancer
Answers: A D

Prostatic cancer is usually an adenocarcinoma and all types of tumour are found from well differentiated to poorly differentiated. This range of differentiation may even be seen within the same tumour. Prostate-specific antigen is an accurate marker of prostate cancer but not a reliable diagnostic investigation because it can be raised in patients with benign hypertrophy. Prostate cancer responds objectively to hormone therapy in about 40% of cases.

SINGLE BEST ANSWER QUESTIONS

1. Childhood urinary tract infection
Answer: E

Although most children come to no harm from urinary tract infection (UTI) the fundamental objective is to identify those at risk of developing permanent renal damage. Diagnosis of UTI usually requires pure urinary culture of 10^5/ml. Childhood urinary tract infection is associated with vesico-ureteric reflux in 2 out of 3 affected children and is caused by an unsuspected surgical disorder in 5% of children. Single antibiotics are usually used for treatment, for example trimethoprim.

2. Breast cancer
Answer: C

Breast cancer is the most common cancer affecting women, with every woman having about a 1 in 10 risk of developing breast cancer in her life. Screening women over 50 years of age may produce a decrease in mortality. Extending the age range of women in the screening programme from 65 to 70 may prevent more deaths. However, shortening the interval from three to two years between screening sessions, may gain more life years. Tamoxifen treatment improves survival by 15–20% with oestrogen receptor positive tumours. Tamoxifen also reduces the incidence of cancer in the other breast. However, the risk of endometrial cancer appears to be increased.

3. Oral contraceptive steroids
Answer: C

Oral contraceptive steroids protect against benign breast disease, carcinoma of the uterus and ovary. The risk of venous thrombosis and pulmonary embolism is related to the oestrogen content of the combined contraceptive pill.

4. Endometrial cancer
Answer: D

Progestogen-based oral contraceptives may have a protective effect against endometrial cancer. Endometrial cancer is usually a well-differentiated adenocarcinoma.

5. Oral contraceptive pill
Answer: D

There is no evidence that progesterone alone increases blood pressure. Even in low dose, the combined oestrogen and progesterone contraceptive pill increases arterial pressure. Established or developing hypertension is therefore a contraindication to a combined pill. Oestrogens increase the risk of arterial or venous thrombosis in some women. The progesterone only preparation appears safe. If a women of over 35 years smokes then the risk of serious cardiovascular events is greatly elevated if she is receiving a combined but not a progesterone only pill. Certain tumours may be oestrogen sensitive e.g. malignant melanoma, hepatoma, desmoid tumours or carcinoma of the breast. As with oestrogens, the metabolism of progesterone is increased by the concurrent use of anticonvulsants that are hepatic enzyme inducers. The combined preparations probably do not enhance the risk of thrombotic crises in sickle cell disease.

6. Bladder cancer
Answer: C

Bladder cancer is usually a transitional cell carcinoma. Most tumours at presentation are superficial. Up to 30% of superficial tumours become invasive, despite adequate treatment. Chemotherapy for metastases improves life expectancy.

7. Prostate cancer
Answer: E

Prostate cancer is the most common cancer in men, and the second commonest cause of cancer death after lung cancer. Over 50% have metastatic spread at diagnosis. Pain is a common feature in the terminal care. Screening results in greatly increased detection but without clear indication of improved survival.

RESPIRATORY MEDICINE

EXTENDED MATCHING QUESTIONS

THEME: BREATHLESSNESS

1. **A** Allergic alveolitis
2. **D** Lung cancer
3. **B** Asthma
4. **F** Pulmonary embolism
5. **E** Myocardial infarction

In clinical scenarios look carefully at the whole scenario searching for key features. Decide on the diagnosis and then look to see if it is in the option list. Look again now at these scenarios with the 'correct' answers in mind. Notice the aviary in the history and the crepitations in the examination of the patient with allergic alveolitis. The female sex and younger age and use of oral contraceptives make diagnosis of pulmonary embolism more likely.

THEME: BREATHLESSNESS

6. **G** Pulmonary fibrosis
7. **A** Pleural effusion
8. **D** Anaemia
9. **E** Pneumothorax
10. **B** Inhalation of foreign body
11. **I** Left ventricular failure

Pulmonary fibrosis may be secondary to inhalation of dust or chemicals, idiopathic, iatrogenic e.g. After radiotherapy, congenital or a pulmonary manifestation of systemic disease e.g. Rheumatoid arthritis. Pleural effusion may be caused by many conditions, including ovarian hyper stimulation syndrome, where it is associated with ascites. Breathlessness may be caused not only by disease of the lungs and heart, and extra thoracic causes should always be considered. Expansion of trapped air in the alveolar tree on ascent may cause alveolar rupture and pneumothorax in scuba divers. This may lead to cerebral arterial gas embolism. For this reason asthmatics (who often have a degree of air trapping) and patients with a history of spontaneous pneumothorax should not dive. Inhalation of foreign bodies may also present sub acutely with signs of localised rhonchi and crepitations if smaller objects pass into the lower bronchi. Left ventricular failure may be precipitated by myocardial infarction, arrhythmias or fluid overload.

MULTIPLE BEST ANSWER QUESTIONS

1. Childhood asthma   Answers: A B

Cough may be the only symptom in some children. Outdoor exercise should not be discouraged. Inhaled steroids are usually used for prevention. They do not normally stunt growth, sodium cromoglycates can be used but is not the drug of choice.

2. Smoking   Answers: A C

GP advice is effective in helping smoking cessation. Nicotine replacement therapy appears to double the rate of smoking cessation achieved by GP advice alone. Many patients will have already thought about their smoking habit and the doctor-patient relationship can be harmed if routine anti-smoking advice is given to all patients. The current increase in smoking is due to the number of younger people starting to smoke. People who have never smoked have a much greater risk of ischaemic heart disease if they live with a smoker.

3. Severe asthma attack   Answers: A C D

Severe asthma is characterised by frequent attacks, limited daily activities, disturbed sleep to 'early morning dips', low PEFR readings (usually 50% or less of normal PEFR readings) and tachycardia. Central cyanosis rather than peripheral cyanosis occurs in severe asthma.

4. Chronic obstructive pulmonary disease   Answers: A C

After standardisation for smoking, men are still more at risk then women of chronic obstructive airways disease. Low socio-economic status is also a risk factor.

5. Lung cancer   Answers: A B E

Lung cancer is most prevalent among people aged over 70 years and causes deaths in the ratio 2:1 for men and women in the UK. It is associated with the level of urban pollution. Adenocarcinoma occurs amongst non-smokers and squamous cell carcinoma among smokers. No genetic association has been clearly established for lung cancer.

6. Increased resonance   Answers: B C D

In pneumothorax and emphysema, the liver may be pushed downwards to give the impression of hepatomegaly.

SINGLE BEST ANSWER QUESTIONS

1. Finger clubbing   Answer: B

Think of pulmonary (bronchiectasis, lung abscess, lung cancer), cardiac (cyanotic congenital heart disease, infective endocarditis) and extra-thoracic (cirrhosis, inflammatory bowel disease) causes. It occurs in empyema rather than emphysema.

2. Inhaled steroids   Answer: B
Some systemic absorption will take place. Inhaled steroid in high dosage may slow growth in children, but side-effects are unusual at low doses. Inhaled steroids are not indicated for use in episodic wheezing. Fluticasone may be less systemically absorbed.

3. Chest infections   Answer: C
Very few chest infections seen in General Practice are due to pneumonia, but of patients with lower respiratory tract infections who receive antibiotics. Antibiotics are of value in an exacerbation of chronic obstructive airways disease.

4. Asthma in children   Answer: D
Skin allergy tests are generally uninformative and should not be ordered routinely. Chest radiographs are only indicated for acute episodes if complications are suspected. Pulmonary function tests become reliable in children aged 7–8 years and over.

5. Recognised causes of cough   Answer: C
Common causes of cough include infections (upper and lower respiratory), postnasal drip, asthma, smoking, lung cancer, inhaled foreign body (especially peanuts), lung diseases (e.g. cystic fibrosis, fibrosing alveolitis) and gastro-oesophageal reflux disease. Consider also medication (ACE inhibitors due to effects on the bradykinin system in the throat), pulmonary oedema ('cardiac asthma'), pertussis and TB.

6. Diagnosis of asthma   Answer: B
Cough is an essential feature in diagnosis, so is family history. Reversibility test is useful, but not essential. 50% of children with asthma are not asthmatic after the age of 7. Steroid inhalers do not have an immediate effect and are for prevention.

7. Bronchial carcinoma   Answer: E
Bronchial carcinoma is now the most common malignant disease in Western Europe. Occupational risk factors include exposure to asbestos, nickel, arsenic, haematite, chromates and radioactivity.

8. Asthma   Answer: D
Asthma mortality has not improved significantly over the past 50 years. Long-acting inhaled bronchodilators are usually recommended when inhaled steroids have provided inadequate control. Viral infections commonly precipitate attacks. Virtually all symptomatic asthmatics have hyperreactive airways, as do a significant number of the normal population. There is no direct adrenergic innervation of the airways. Beta-2 agonists act on adrenergic receptors.

ADMINISTRATION
AND MANAGEMENT
ANSWERS

EXTENDED MATCHING QUESTIONS

THEME: LEGISLATION

1. **E** Rehabilitation of Offenders Act 1974
2. **B** Access to Medical Reports Act 1988
3. **A** Access to Health Records Act 1990
4. **D** Disability Discrimination Act 1995
5. **C** Data Protection Act 1984

You need to know some of the background about these Acts.
Data Protection Act 1984 – controls computer-held personal data
Rehabilitation of Offenders Act 1974 – results in certain convictions being 'spent'
Disability Discrimination Act 1995 – gives employers duties in relation to employees with present or past disabilities
Access to Health Records Act 1990 – allows patients access to their own medical notes
Access to Medical Reports Act 1988 – allows patients to see reports

THEME: VOLUNTARY ORGANISATIONS

6. **J** RNIB
7. **D** CRUSE
8. **I** RELATE
9. **G** MIND
10. **M** Terrence Higgins Trust
11. **C** Compassionate Friends
12. **A** Alanon
13. **H** NSPCC
14. **E** Gingerbread
15. **F** Marie Curie Memorial Foundation
16. **D** CRUSE
17. **B** ASH
18. **N** Turning point

There are many voluntary organisations. You should at least know what they are concerned with:
RNIB – Blindness
CRUSE – Widows with bereavement problems and children suffering bereavement problems after death of parents
RELATE – Marriage problems
MIND – Mental illness
Terrence Higgins Trust – AIDS
Compassionate Friends – Bereaved parents
Alanon – Relatives of people with alcohol problems
NSPCC – Child abuse
Gingerbread – One parent families

Marie Curie Memorial Foundation – Cancer
ASH – Smokers
Turning Point – Drug abuse

THEME: MEDICAL CERTIFICATES

19.	**D**	Med 6
20.	**A**	Med 3
21.	**D**	Med 6
22.	**F**	DS 1500
23.	**B**	Med 4
24.	**A**	Med 3
25.	**C**	Med 5

All medical practitioners need to know about certification for sickness absence. Med 3 is the usual sickness certificate – the patient must be seen, and this certificate can initially be issued for up to six months. Med 4 is only issued when the personal capability incapacity test is being considered. Med 5 is issued when a patient was seen previously or there is a recent medical report about the patient. Med 6 is to be used when a vague diagnosis has deliberately been put on another certificate – usually in the interests of confidentiality. Hospital personnel issue Med 10. A DS 1500 is issued when a patient has a terminal illness and has applied for Disability Living Allowance or Attendance Allowance.

THEME: REGULATORY BODIES

26.	**C**	National Institute for Clinical Excellence
27.	**E**	National Clinical Assessment Authority
28.	**G**	Primary Care Trust
29.	**F**	United Kingdom Central Council (UKCC)
30.	**B**	Joint Committee for Post Graduate Training in General Practice

The UKCC is the nursing equivalent of the GMC. Local medical committees are the local representatives of general practitioners in a particular area. The Commission for Health Improvement is charged with inspecting health facilities to ensure they meet certain minimum standards.

THEME: NUMBERS OF PEOPLE ON A GP'S LIST

31.	**E**	100
32.	**A**	5
33.	**C**	25
34.	**F**	200
35.	**B**	10

You need to have a good idea about the frequency of events and the occurrence of diseases. In an average GP list, there will be 5 schizophrenics, 10 blind people, 25 deaf people, 100 unemployed people and 200 people on state benefits.

THEME: GP INCOME

36. **E** Registration fees
37. **I** Immunisation item of service fees
38. **K** Temporary resident fee
39. **L** Emergency treatment fee
40. **C** Immediately necessary treatment fee

The rules governing payments for patients not on your list are complex. For stays in the area less than 24 hours or for patients unable to reach their own GP an Emergency Treatment form is used. For patients refused acceptance onto full list or as temporary resident Immediately necessary treatment forms are used. For patients in the area for more than 24 hours but less than three months who are accepted as temporary residents this form is used. If a request is made and a face-to-face consultation occurs after 10 pm an additional night visit fee is paid. Temporary resident claims may include telephone consultations. In exceptional circumstances, e.g. a new partner inheriting a large list, the three month period for new patient registrations may be extended to two years.

MULTIPLE BEST ANSWER QUESTIONS

1.   Seizures   Answers: A D E
The patient but not his or her doctor is obliged to contact the DVLA, although it is sensible practice to record in the case notes that a patient has been counselled about driving. Patients must be free from any attack for two years or have had only attacks whilst asleep for three years before driving is permitted. A diagnosis of primary malignant cerebral tumour, cerebral metastasis or even bronchogenic carcinoma without cerebral metastasis is associated with such a high risk of a seizure that driving is prohibited.

2.   History of epilepsy   Answers: B C
Teachers in training have to have been seizure-free for two years. Similarly, a recent history would be a problem as a prison officer. Any history of epilepsy would be a barrier for employment as aircraft pilots, train drivers and army officers. Merchant seafarers must not have had a fit since the age of 5 years.

3.   Burnout in General Practitioners   Answers: B D E
Burnout appears to be a response to stress and dissatisfaction. There is a relation to depressive illness. Obsessional, idealistic and conscientious doctors, who are reluctant to delegate, are more likely to get burnt out. Fortunately, attendance at postgraduate meetings and postgraduate qualifications seem to have a protective influence against burnout.

4. Heartsink patients   Answers: C D E
Postgraduate qualifications and counselling training appear to reduce the number of patients seen or perceived as heartsink patients. Lower job satisfaction and a greater number of heartsink patients are related, but it is unclear which is cause or effect. About 1/3 have a serious medical diagnosis of some sort and non-attendance at appointments is high.

5. Over-the-counter medicine   Answers: A C D
Medicines should be POM if they are normally administered by injection, if they are new and need further investigation, if they are frequently used incorrectly and if they are dangerous if used other than under medical supervision. Cimetidine has been over-the-counter (OTC) from 1993 while ibuprofen has been available since 1983 and topical acyclovir since 1993. Piroxicam is only available OTC in topical version (since 1994).

6. Free NHS prescriptions   Answers: B D E
Patients with myxoedema or conditions requiring supplemental thyroxine get free prescriptions, as do some thyrotoxics needing concomitant thyroxine. Diabetics on diet alone do not get free prescriptions. Free prescriptions are available to patients with permanent fistula e.g caecostomy, colostomy, laryngostomy or ileostomy needing continuous surgical dressing or appliance. Also, patients with hypoparathyroidism, hypopituitarism or continuing physical disability needing the help of another person. Don't forget free prescriptions for pregnant women.

7. Advance directives   Answers: B C D
An advance directive can be revoked if the patient requests and is competent to make that request. There is a need to be explicit about the possibility of death in the directive, which needs to be signed and witnessed. The advance directive must not be deliberately ignored. Very basic care including hydration and nutrition will be maintained.

8. Terms of Service for GPs   Answers: A C D
The 26 hours will include visiting but not 'on call' time. There is a clause allowing certain doctors (e.g. those involved in teaching) to be available only four days a week but they must be available 42 weeks out of 52 weeks. The 24–hour responsibility can be delegated to a deputising service or a 'co-op'. The 'items of service' payments need to be claimed for but capitation payments are made with respect to Health Authority figures of list size. However, one can dispute the figures for capitation. Cervical smears are paid on reaching targets (i.e. 50% and 80% being the 'targets' for smears).

9. Items of Service payments   Answers: C D E
Cervical smears are 'target' payments as are childhood immunisations but GPs are paid for some vaccinations (e.g. tetanus, travel, etc). The 'old' FP1001 for contraception advice is now on a multi-claim form GMS4, as are night visit claims. Maternity work is claimed on GMS2 forms.

10. Confirmation of death **Answers: A B E**

Reportable deaths are where the cause is unknown, unnatural cause, abortion, suicide, industrial disease, due to medication, drugs or poisons, deaths due to injury, not seen by a medical practitioner in the last illness or not seen in the last 14 days.

11. Personal Medical Services **Answers: B C D**

In essence PMS is a reformulation of the provision of General Medical Services, but allows the Government to cash limit AND to transfer some element of secondary care to primary care. In the GMS system, GPs claim for each 'Items of Service' done and the Government does not know in advance how much the GP will claim in that year. PMS aims to:

1. Reduce bureaucracy (no individual Items of Service claims) within the Health Service. Doctors are bound by the contract they sign. Also, since they work under contract, there is no security of the level that the Red Book provides to GPs.
2. Transfer increasing secondary care to primary care
3. Limit cash
4. Give increased autonomy to GPs
5. Allow for salaried GPs

12. Principal in General Practice **Answers: D E**

A principal is responsible for assistants, locums, nurses and others who deal with patients registered under their name; and they are responsible to these patients 24 hours a day seven days a week. They have to receive a one-third share of the partner with the greatest share. To get postgraduate allowance, they have to do five days of approved study. They do get an automatic seniority allowance.

13. General Practice premises **Answers: C E**

Most General Practitioners work in owner-occupied premises, for which they receive a notional or cost rent. All public buildings have to meet the requirements of the Disability Act. They can use the premises for private work, but income cannot exceed 10% of total income. The rent is reviewed by the District Valuer every three years.

14. Red book **Answers: A C**

A quality payment is paid to all training practices. Other practices have to meet certain quality criteria, including having notes in chronological order. The Prescribing Incentive Scheme is not part of the red book and is generally locally negotiated. The assistance allowance is based on list size, but retainees are not and they can now work for up to four sessions. Minor surgery payments are based on number of principals, but not on list size.

15. Prescription on FP10   Answers: A B D

Viagra can be prescribed in a limited group; patients outside this category can only be given private treatment. Paracetamol can be given, but not as Panadol. Neck collars can be obtained from hospitals, but not on FP10.

16. Patient records   Answers: C E

Paper records are the property of the Secretary of State. A patient may include a statement contesting the report but may not insist on it being amended. Third party details may be disguised to protect individuals. Practices may make a reasonable charge for access to any records.

SINGLE BEST ANSWER

1. Commercial flights   Answer: B

Most commercial flights will allow pregnant women of up to 34 weeks gestational age to be carried on board.

2. GP Service Contract   Answer: B

The core General Medical Services Contract covers most of the General Practitioner's work, which includes provision of a statutory sick note after seven days of absence from work. The Family Planning Service requires a separate contract and attracts an additional fee. There is no provision for annual health checks. There is, however, limited provision for minor surgery, but not as a core activity and therefore attracts a fee. The core contract expects a letter of invitation for a health check to all over 75.

3. Computerised Medical Records   Answer: C

From August 2000, it became legal not to have paper records, and Items of Service links are now widely used in most General Practices. There has not been any good research study to show that computers hinder consultations. There is, however, good evidence to show that nurses are better at data entry with regards to templates. The evidence from computers can be used and was indeed what led to conviction for Dr Shipman.

4. Personal Medical Services (PMS)   Answer: B

Personal medical services pilots were introduced in 1997, to allow greater flexibility in the provision of General Practice services. They allowed employment of salaried doctors and the employment could be by nurses, GPs or Community Trusts. The PMS only contract does not include prescribing or provision of secondary care services, but PMS+ can allow for this.

5. Mental Health Act   Answer: B

Section 3 is the most appropriate section to use for a patient with an established psychiatric diagnosis who has to be admitted compulsorily for treatment.

6.   General Medical Council   **Answer: C**
The General Medical Council has recently revised its guidance to doctors and these
are published as five separate booklets. Most of the information is covered under
duties of the doctor. Doctors do not have to meet performance targets set by
management if they disagree with them, but if non-provision of the targets can be
shown to cause harm to patients, the doctor would have a very weak case.

7.   NHS Direct   **Answer: B**
Although this service is planned to be available all over the country, it has not been
fully evaluated and not shown to be cost effective. It is usually run by nurses. Legal
cover has to be provided, as there is no Crown immunity for the service.

8.   PGEA   **Answer: D**
25 days CME spread over five years entitles the principal to full payment. VTS
training counts for the first year only. CME may be distance learning, consultant
supervision, taught courses, by assessment of personal learning plans or internet-
based tutorials.

9.   Financing for premises   **Answer: D**
Cost rent involves rent at a rate linked to base rates at the time of entering the
agreement being paid by the FHSA, while partners pay off the capital. The FHSA
rate is fixed, but the finance may be changed to take advantage of falling interest
rates. When the value of the property increases the practice may change from cost
rent to notional rent. PMS contracts make provision for development of green field
sites only.

10.   Drugs carried in a GP's bag   **Answer: C**
Under the terms of service a GP must keep a supply of drugs to administer in
emergencies. These must not be replaced with FP 10 prescribed drugs in the
patient's name. Controlled drugs must be kept in a locked car boot; a locked car is
insufficient. A dispensing fee is payable for all drugs administered to all patients.

11.   Complaints   **Answer: E**
There must be a nominated person and a deputy to administer the system, but
these may be anyone in the practice. There must be an acknowledgement within
two working days and a response within 10. The time limit to lodge a complaint is
one year. 90% of complaints are due to failure to visit, examine, diagnose or refer.

RESEARCH, EPIDEMIOLOGY AND STATISTICS ANSWERS

EXTENDED MATCHING QUESTIONS

THEME: XENICAL

1.	**K**	30
2.	**J**	28
3.	**T**	Hypertension
4.	**C**	2.5
5.	**P**	Dietary
6.	**R**	Activity
7.	**E**	5
8.	**F**	6
9.	**G**	10
10.	**A**	1
11.	**B**	2

Xenical (Orlistat) is a pancreatic lipase inhibitor. It helps weight loss by impairing uptake of fats in the gut. It has no effect on uptake of calories in any other form, so patients must lose weight by a reduction in calorie intake. It may lead to faecal incontinence if fats are consumed and potentially may lead to a deficiency of fat-soluble vitamins A,D,E and K.

THEME: STATISTICS

12.	**B**	112/175
13.	**A**	112/183
14.	**J**	754/817
15.	**K**	754/825

However the way the question is presented, it is best to write out the figures in a table:

	Disease present	Disease absent	Total
Test positive	112	71	183
Test negative	63	754	817
Total	175	825	1000

Then:

Sensitivity = 112/175
Specificity = 754/825
Positive predictive value = 112/183
Negative predictive value = 754/817

THEME: TRIALS

16. **D** Descriptive study
17. **A** Case control study
18. **F** Randomised clinical trial
19. **C** Correlation study
20. **E** Meta-analysis study

You need to be clear about the types of trials and studies. Remember that:

- Cohort studies follow forward groups, otherwise matched, with different exposures to the topic of concern.
- Case control studies compare patients with the disease/problem with controls looking at past exposure/events.
- Correlation looks for an association between quantitative variables.

THEME: STATISTICAL TERMS

21. **E** 2
22. **E** 2
23. **E** 2

It is best to put the numbers in order:
0,0,1,1,1,2,2,2,2,4,7.
The average (mean) is 22/11 = 2
The median (in the middle) is 2
The mode (most common) is 2

THEME: ECONOMICS

24. **B** Cost benefit analysis
25. **A** Cost
26. **F** Cost effectiveness ratio
27. **H** Cost of illness analysis
28. **I** Cost utility analysis

A cost benefit analysis is a type of economic assessment in which both cost and benefit are expressed in monetary terms. Cost is the monetary value of the resources consumed in its production or delivery. Cost effectiveness ratio is the ratio of total cost of an intervention divided by the gain in selected health outcome. Cost of illness analysis estimates the economic burden of a particular disease. Cost utility analysis assesses the benefit of an intervention.

THEME: STUDIES

29. **B** Cohort study
30. **F** Randomised double blind cross-over trial
31. **G** Randomised double blind placebo-controlled trial
32. **A** Case control study
33. **D** Descriptive

Think about the types of trials and studies. Remember that:
Cohort studies are prospective studies following matched groups with different exposures to the subject of concern. Case control studies are retrospective studies comparing patients with the disease/problem with controls and looking at past exposure/events. Correlation looks for an association between quantitative variables. Descriptive studies often simply describe what has been found, or what prevalence of a disease has been noted.

THEME: SCREENING TESTS

34. **H** 80%
35. **I** 93%
36. **D** 25%
37. **B** 0.8
38. **C** 20%

	Disease	No disease
Test positive	A (20)	B (5)
Test negative	C (5)	D (70)

Sensitivity –	A sensitive test detects a high proportion of the true cases – measured here by $a/(a + c)$.
Specificity –	A highly specific test has very few false positives – measured by $d/(b +d)$.
Systematic error –	This is measured by the ratio of the total numbers positive to the test and those with the disease, or $(a + b)/(a + c)$.
Prevalence –	$a+c/(a+b+c+d)$
Predictive value –	This is the proportion of positive test results that are truly positive – measured as $a/(a+b)$. It is important in screening.
Yield –	$a/(a+b+c+d)$

Systematic error, yield and predictive value depend on the relative frequency of true positives and true negatives in the study sample (i.e. on the prevalence of the disease or exposure that is being measured).

THEME: RESEARCH METHODS

39. **A** Clinical audit
40. **F** Survey
41. **D** Qualitative study
42. **E** Randomised controlled trial
43. **B** Longitudinal study

These are examples of research methods now used in General Practice. The explanation is generally in the answer. Other studies may be used for some of the answers, but most likely answers are expected.

THEME: STATISTICAL TERMS

44. **B** Sensitivity analysis
45. **E** Standard deviation
46. **A** Sensitivity
47. **F** Standard error of the mean (SEM)
48. **H** Standardised mortality rate

Common definitions to common terms used in research papers. There is an expectation that you are familiar with these terms.

THEME: LITERATURE IN GENERAL PRACTICE

49. **B** Pendleton D, *The consultation*, Oxford, 1984.
50. **A** Stott CP, Davis RH, *The exceptional potential in each primary care consultation*. JRCGP 1979; 29: 201–5.
51. **F** Byrne PS, Long BEL, *Doctors talking to patients*, DHSS, 1976.
52. **E** Balint M, *The doctor, his patient and the illness*, London Tavistock, 1958.
53. **B** Pendleton D, *The consultation*, Oxford, 1984.
54. **C** Berne E, *Transactional analysis – Games people play*, Penguin, 1970.
55. **D** Heron J, *Human potential research project*, Univ of Surrey, 1975.
56. **A** Stott CP, Davis RH, *The exceptional potential in each primary care consultation*. JRCGP 1979; 29: 201–5.
57. **G** Neighbour R, *The Inner Consultation*, Petroc Press, 1999.
58. **E** Balint M, *The doctor, his patient and the illness*, London Tavistock, 1958.

You need to be familiar with General Practice literature. Pendleton's 'The Consultation' discussed seven tests and discussed achieving a shared understanding with the patient. Balink's 'The Doctor his patient and the illness' describes both the apostolic function of the doctor, and the use of the doctor as a 'drug'.

THEME: A YEAR IN GENERAL PRACTICE

59. **E** <1
60. **A** 500

61. B 200
62. D 10
63. C 25

You need to have a good idea about the frequency of events and the occurrence of diseases.

In an average year in an average General Practice, about 500 people consult because of chronic mental illness, about 200 because of hypertension, about 25 because of diabetes, about 10 with a thyroid problem, and less than 1 with chronic renal failure.

THEME: TRIALS CONCERNING CORONARY HEART DISEASE

64. D GISSI
65. E GREAT Group Study
66. A 4S
67. C CARE Study
68. F ISIS-2
69. G Nurses Study
70. B ASSET

Important trials of thrombolytic therapy include ISIS-2, GISSI and ASSET. ISIS-2 involved treating patients with streptokinase and/or aspirin. GISSI involved streptokinase and placebo. ASSET used alteplase.

The GREAT Group Study was about the pre-hospital treatment of patients using anistreplase as the active drug.

Two large-scale drug trials using lipid lowering drugs on people needing secondary prevention were 4S and CARE Study. 4S used simvastatin; CARE used pravastatin therapy. The Nurses study of unopposed oestrogen showed a large reduction in the incidence of ischaemic heart disease.

THEME: CARDIOVASCULAR TRIALS

71. F WOSCOPS
72. A SOLVD-T
73. G CARE
74. E ISIS-2
75. I HOT
76. B UKPDS-1998

The HOT trial confirmed that the lowest incidence of cardiovascular complications occurred at a diastolic BP of 82.6 mmHg. 4S looked at secondary prevention in patients with hypercholesterolaemia. HOPE confirmed the value of ramipril in high-risk patients. The antiplatelet trialists collaboration 94 demonstrated the benefit of aspirin 75 mg a day for secondary prevention. UKPDS 1998 in particular demonstrated the value of tight BP control in diabetes but also confirmed the value of metformin.

THEME: HYPERTENSION

77. **F** Non-pharmacological measures
78. **B** 100
79. **H** 15
80. **C** 145
81. **J** 85
82. **D** 150
83. **K** 90
84. **O** Thiazides
85. **Q** Beta blockers
86. **P** Aspirin
87. **T** Statins

The general principles of hypertension are to confirm the diagnosis with at least three separate readings, try lifestyle measures first, such as weight loss and exercise, then start treatment with low dose thiazides or beta blockers. The choice of second line agent will depend on the patient; diabetics should be treated with ACE inhibitors, while these are relatively ineffective in blacks and the elderly. The full guidance can be found at www.hyp.ac.uk

MULTIPLE BEST ANSWER QUESTIONS

1.   Mental health of children and adolescents   Answers: A D E
10% of children between 5 and 15 years have a significant mental disorder, with boys being particularly affected. Children in families without a working parent are particularly vulnerable in this respect. Almost 50% of children with a mental disorder will have been seen by their GP that year but 30% have no contact with a GP or specialist service. The proportion of children with special educational needs is three times higher in children with a mental disorder.

2.   Children   Answers: A D
Infant mortality in Social Class V is very much higher than that in Social Class I. Children in Social Class V are more likely to die in an accident; they have twice the rate of chronic illness and they are shorter.

3.   Obesity in the UK   Answers: A E
The prevalence of obesity is increasing in most of the western world and is more common in people from lower social economic class. Medical means of treatment should only be used with BMI >30 and the patients show motivation by losing weight themselves. The South Asian population has a different hip to waist ratio and may have risk of heart disease despite normal BMI. Loss of weight in obese patients would result in reduction of blood pressure.

4. Liver cirrhosis   Answers: B C

Publicans, boatmen, hotel managers, fishermen, chefs and journalists, are some of the groups most likely to die from liver cirrhosis. 10 years ago doctors had 300% greater than average risk of dying from cirrhosis, but recently this figure has dropped hugely.

5. NSF on Cardiovascular disease   Answers: C D E

NSF on CHD was published in March 2000 and includes targets for health and social care, including local authorities. Specialist smoking cessation clinics are recommended but not in General Practice setting. There are specific targets for revascularisation, disease registers and cardiac rehabilitation.

6. Retrospective studies   Answers: A C D

In retrospective studies great stress is placed on memory and past history; bias is very common. They are cheaper to carry out and take a shorter time to conduct.

7. Trials   Answers: B C E

The chi-squared tests is a non-parametric test (data grouped by category) which is always carried out on absolute numbers not proportions, means or percentages. The method is to construct a table using the data, then for each cell the expected number is calculated. The difference between the observed and expected is recorded, the result squared and dived by the expected number $[(O-E)^2/E]$; the chi-squared statistic is the sum of all the values. The degree of freedom is (number of rows – 1) multiplied by (number of columns – 1). Potential confounding variables occur where there is some factor, other than the one you are testing, influencing the result.

8. Systematic reviews   Answers: A B E

Systematic reviews refers to the systematic, quantitative, pooling of available randomised controlled trials. The results of meta-analysis are usually presented graphically, with confidence intervals (typically 95%). They are not available for most medical interventions as RCTs are not available and commissioners are generally not in a position to use these in making decisions.

Poor RCT studies can produce wrong conclusions, as these will be compounded by pooled estimates of effect.

9. Studies   Answers: C D

The prevalence of condition reflects the total number of cases in a population at a given time.

Cohort studies may be used to study a defined group through time e.g. a group of subjects exposed to a suspected cause of a disease at a particular time are then followed up to see whether they develop the disease.

The mode is the value which occurs most frequently i.e. the maximum value on the frequency distribution curve. If a distribution is positively skewed with a long tail on the right side and more large values, the mode will be less than the mean. Similarly, if the distribution is negatively skewed (long tail on the left, more small values) the mode will be greater than the mean.

The standard error of the mean of a sample (SEM) is a measure of how accurately the true population mean has been estimated. It may be calculated by dividing the standard deviation of the sample by the square root of the sample size (SD/square root of n).

10. Standard deviation   Answers: B C D
The standard deviation is a measure of the scatter of observations about the mean. It is distorted by extreme values when compared to the range. Standard deviation is the square root of the variance. The standard error is a measure of the accuracy of the sample mean when compared with the unknown population mean. It is calculated by SD/ (square root of N), where N is the number in the sample. The chi-squared tests is a non-parametric test and is carried out on absolute numbers not proportions, means or percentages.

11. Statistics   Answers: B C D
p = 0.001 means that the results could have occurred by chance at 1 in a 100 observations, p = 0.05 occurs in 1 in 20 observations. The former is of greater statistical significance. Prevalence is the total number of cases (old and new) at a certain point in time. The incidence is the number of new cases occurring over a set period. In a chronic condition prevalence is much greater than incidence. In a short-lived condition prevalence can equal incidence. The mean is the average value, the mode the most frequently occurring value and the median the value in the middle.

12. Study   Answers: A C E
The mean and standard deviation should completely define the normal distribution, with 95% of the sample data lying within an interval defined by the mean +/- 2 standard deviations. The variance is the square of the standard deviation.
In any study it is hoped that the sample mean will be equal to the population mean, but they are most unlikely to be exactly equal. Remember that the median is equal to the mean when the data are normally distributed.

13. Study   Answers: C E
Statistical significance does not imply clinical significance. In addition to assessing the clinical improvement produced by a therapy, account must also be taken of side-effects.

Chi-squared is a calculated statistic used to compare proportions and has no immediate intuitive meaning unlike a p-value or a mean. Any bias or confounding element (e.g. differences in the severity of disease between the two groups) may invalidate a trial.

14. Clinical trial of a new treatment   Answers: B C D

The null hypothesis is rejected if there is a significant difference between the groups. A type I error occurs when the null hypothesis is wrongly rejected (i.e. concluding that a significant difference exists when in reality it does not). A type II error occurs when the null hypothesis is accepted when in reality a genuine difference exists between the two groups.

The power of a trial is the probability of rejecting the null hypothesis when it is false i.e. of concluding a difference or result of a given size is statistically significant. The power of a trial generally is increased when the number of participants is large and is decreased if the difference to be detected is small.

15. Correlation methods   Answers: A C

Correlation methods are used to examine whether there is a linear relationship between two continuous variables; the strength of the association is reflected in the value of r from -1 to +1.

If the correlation is strong r has values of less than –0.5 or greater than +0.5. The statistical significance of a particular r is calculated separately. Even if a correlation is poor, it may still be statistically significant. Although two variables may be correlated, this does not allow a value for one variable to be calculated from a value of the second. Regression analysis and the derivation of a regression equation may be used to calculate the value of one (dependent) variable from a second (independent) variable. Mortality is not a continuous variable.

16. Mean   Answers: B C D

Normal distribution is not the only symmetrical distribution; many other symmetrical distributions exist. If the observations had been found to be positively skewed, their mode would have been less than the mean. The median time is equal to the 50th percentile. The variance of the observations would provide a measure of their spread about the mean. The standard error is a measure of the reliability of the mean value.

17. Referral rates   Answers: A B

Referral rate appears to be related to the individual doctor and not to the prescribing pattern or the size of the practice. Deprivation accounts for about one-third of the variation. GP experience in a particular field can actually increase the referral rate.

18. GPs patients   Answers: B D E

(From J.Fry, *General Practice – the facts*.)

Condition	Persons consulting per year per 2000
Acute bronchitis	116
Pneumonia	12
Acute myocardial infarction	8
(sudden death)	(4)
Acute stroke	6
Severe depression	10
(parasuicide)	(4)

Suicide	(1 in 4 years)
Acute abdominal conditions	6
All new cancers	8

19. The Oxcheck Study   Answers: C D
The Oxcheck study was a study of primary prevention in coronary heart disease. It looked at nurse-led risk factor intervention clinics in the General Practice setting. The clinics were expensive and the outcome measures showed disappointing results. However, the focus was usefully moved to secondary prevention.

20. UK Prospective Diabetes Study Group   Answers: A B D
The UK Prospective Diabetes Study Group was a very large study. It showed that intensive blood sugar control reduces microvascular complications. The beneficial effects of metformin were noted especially in overweight patients. Metformin reduced mortality from all causes and from diabetic related diseases. Less weight gain was noted with metformin than other treatment regimes. The combination of metformin with a sulphonylurea appeared to be related to an increased mortality. Good control of blood pressure reduced mortality from all causes and from diabetic related causes.

SINGLE BEST ANSWER QUESTIONS

1. Strokes   Answer: A
Strokes are very common and indeed are the commonest cause of disability. They are the second most common cause of death in the UK. Each episode of stroke has 30% mortality with a 10% recurrence rate in the first year. 20% are due to haemorrhage, 80% are due to infarction.

2. Hypertension Society guidelines   Answer: A
The British Hypertension Society guidelines were published in 1999; they make use of individual risk assessment. They are based on the prevention of events rather than just on the lowering of blood pressure. The guidelines suggest that all patients should receive non-drug advice, and that optimal levels after treatment are <150/<90 as a minimal acceptable level. The guidelines recognise that these targets will not be achieved in many patients even though most patients will require more than one drug.

3. British Hypertension Society Guidelines   Answer: A
The BHS guidelines recommends annual review at reading of 138/88, but this is not generally practical. The optimal control is <140/<85 mmHg. Patients over 80 should be treated in the same manner as aged 65 and cost benefit is greater. Treatment should generally be started after three readings.

4. Study   Answer: B
A correlation coefficient is a measure of a linear relationship between two independently measured variables. It does not indicate a definite relationship. A

value of 1.0 indicates a perfect positive relationship, -1.0 a negative one and zero the absence of a linear one. It is possible that in a 'U' shaped relationship then the correlation could be zero. The p value depends on the correlation found and the number studied.

5.   Normal (Gaussian) distribution   Answer: D
In a normal distribution the mode is the most frequent observation, the median divides the distribution exactly into two halves; the mean, median and the mode are numerically the same.

A poisson distribution is discrete and relates to the number of events which happen in a fixed time interval. It can be used, for example, to compare death rates that can be regarded as happening by random event in a community.

6.   Median   Answer: C
The median and mode are used in preference to the arithmetic mean when a set of values is from a population with a skewed distribution. In such situations values from the long tail of the skew distribution disproportionately affect the value of the arithmetic mean (average) which may be misleading.

7.   Study   Answer: C
r is simply the correlation coefficient. There is a positive association between the two variables. A statistically significant correlation does not necessarily imply a causal relationship. The small value of p implies that the mathematical relationship present has been established as statistically significant, so more than sufficient infants were studied.

8.   UK respiratory diseases   Answer: A
In the UK respiratory diseases account for 20% of deaths and over 30% of sickness absence from work. 25% of medical admissions to hospital are due to respiratory diseases.

9.   Wheelchair use   Answer: A
Over 20% of wheelchairs are provided for patients with arthritis.

10.   Intermittent claudication   Answer B
Many patients with intermittent claudication find that their symptoms remain static or even improve following presentation, particularly in the first two years. The clinical course is more benign in women than in men. Regular exercise improves blood flow in the long term and should be encouraged. Life expectancy is shorter than in unaffected individuals.

11.   Data from the Framingham Study   Answer: D
The Framingham Study was a large American study of coronary artery disease involving about 5000 people. It was a study of primary prevention and risk factors. The data can be transferred to predict risk in the white population of the UK. However, the data do not apply to those with familial hyperlipidaemia who should be assessed as high risk in any case.

INDEX

Tumours, infective agents 43
Turner's syndrome 44

UK Prospective Diabetes Study
    Group 124
Urinary tract infections 83

Venous leg ulcers 17
Vision, sudden loss of 23
Visual field defects 25

Visual fundus findings 27
Voluntary organisations 93

Warfarin 57, 58
Wheelchair use 126
Wilson's disease 32

Xenical 106

Zanamivir 58

PASTEST REVISION COURSE

MRCGP

All PasTest MRCGP courses are PGEA Approved

Preparing you fully for the exam

PasTest has been helping doctors to pass their exams for the past 30 years. Our extensive experience and network of advisers means that we are always one step ahead of other course providers and publishers when it comes to knowledge of the current trends and content of the exam.

PasTest has been busy preparing for the revised exam format by creating a bank of new style questions, written by a team of Consultants and SpRs, then revised, selected and compiled by our lectures.

The widest range of dates and locations for courses

We recognise that the revision needs and study leave of each candidate differs, we therefore offer a variety of course options to suit individual requirements.

Dynamic and knowledgeable lecturers

Most of our lecturers are Royal College examiners, providing you with the ultimate advantage. With many years membership experience, the tutors have intimate knowledge of the exam and adjust their teaching to reflect the current trends. Throughout the course, they provide valuable tips about exam technique. We constantly evaluate our lecturers through feedback from candidates to ensure that our courses are continually improved.

Impressive pre-course material

Exclusive course notes are provided, including sample questions based on Paper 1 and Paper 2, with diagrams, lists, mnemonics and revision checklists. During the course you will receive correct answers and teaching notes, written by our team of MRCGP question writers.

Course content 100% relevant to the exam

All our MRCGP courses consist of modular sessions, which provide intensive practice of the key elements of the exam. The course is designed to mirror the modular format of the MRCGP EXAMINATION.

The course content includes sessions dedicated to Papers 1 and 2, where you will receive model answers and detailed feedback on the extensive pre-course material. In addition, our tutors will provide invaluable advice on the topics that are likely to appear in the current exam as well as hints and tips on exam technique.

To prepare you for the Oral examination, the College Examiners will provide an insight into what the examiners are looking for. You will then be divided into small groups to practise your technique. You will also receive expert advice, hints and tips on consultation skills to ensure you receive the most complete preparation.

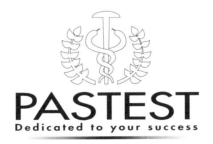

PASTEST
Dedicated to your success

PasTest Ltd, FREEPOST, Knutsford, WA16 7BR.

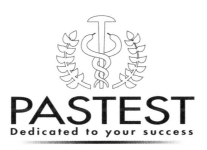

PASTEST
Dedicated to your success

PasTest has been publishing books for doctors for over 30 years. Our extensive experience means that we are always one step ahead when it comes to knowledge of current trends and content of the Royal College exams.

We use only the best authors and lecturers, many of whom are Consultants and Royal College Examiners, which enables us to tailor our books and courses to meet your revision needs. We incorporate feedback from candidates to ensure that our books are continually improved.

This commitment to quality ensures that students who buy a PasTest book or attend a PasTest course achieve successful exam results.

100% Money Back Guarantee
We're sure you will find our study books invaluable, but in the unlikely event that you are not entirely happy, we will give you your money back – guaranteed.

Delivery to your Door
With a busy lifestyle, nobody enjoys walking to the shops for something that may or may not be in stock. Let us take the hassle and deliver direct to your door. We will despatch your book within 24 hours of receiving your order. We also offer free delivery on books for medical students to UK addresses.

How to Order:

www.pastest.co.uk
To order books safely and securely online, shop online at our website.

(Telephone: +44 (0)1565 752000
Fill out the order form as a helpful prompt and have your credit card to hand when you call.

PasTest Ltd, FREEPOST, Knutsford, WA16 7BR.
Send your completed order form with your cheque (made payable to **PasTest Ltd**) and debit or credit card details to the above address. (Please complete your address details on the reverse of the cheque.)

+44 (0)1565 650264
Fax your completed order form with your debit or credit card details.

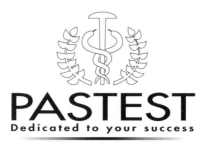

PASTEST REVISION BOOKS

MRCGP Practice Papers: MCQs and EMQs Second edition
P Ellis and P Elliott 1 901198 29 4
- Five complete MCQ and EMQ Practice Papers
- Answers and detailed teaching notes
- Expert advice on successful exam technique
- Comprehensive Revision Index for easy reference to specific topics
- Invaluable intensive practice material for all MRCGP candidates

MRCGP: Approaching the Modular Examination – 2ⁿᵈ edition
L Newson & J Sandars 1 901198 91 X
- Revised and updated to reflect the current modular exam format
- Covers all components of the new exam
- Multiple Choice questions sections with answers and teaching notes
- Critical Appraisal questions based on recent BMJ articles
- Tips on tackling the Audit section
- Relevant for doctors taking the Summative Assessment examination

Practice Papers for the DCH Examination
J Lynch 1 901198 52 9
- Three complete practice papers
- 180 MCQs, 30 Short Note questions and 6 case commentaries
- Section on tackling the Clinical Components
- Comprehensive MCQ Revision Index

DRCOG Practice Exams: MCQs and OSCEs
M Dooley & M Read 1 901198 44 4
- Two complete MCQ Practice Exams with answers and detailed teaching notes
- Twenty OSCE questions with model answers
- Written by two Royal College examiners
- Invaluable Revision Checklist covering the complete syllabus
- Expert advice on exam technique

To order: For 24 hour despatch call 01565 752000 or order books safely and securely online, shop at our website www.pastest.co.uk